The Comprehensive Vegetarian Dish Cookbook

Easy Vegetarian Meal Ideas For Everyone

Lucas Pearson

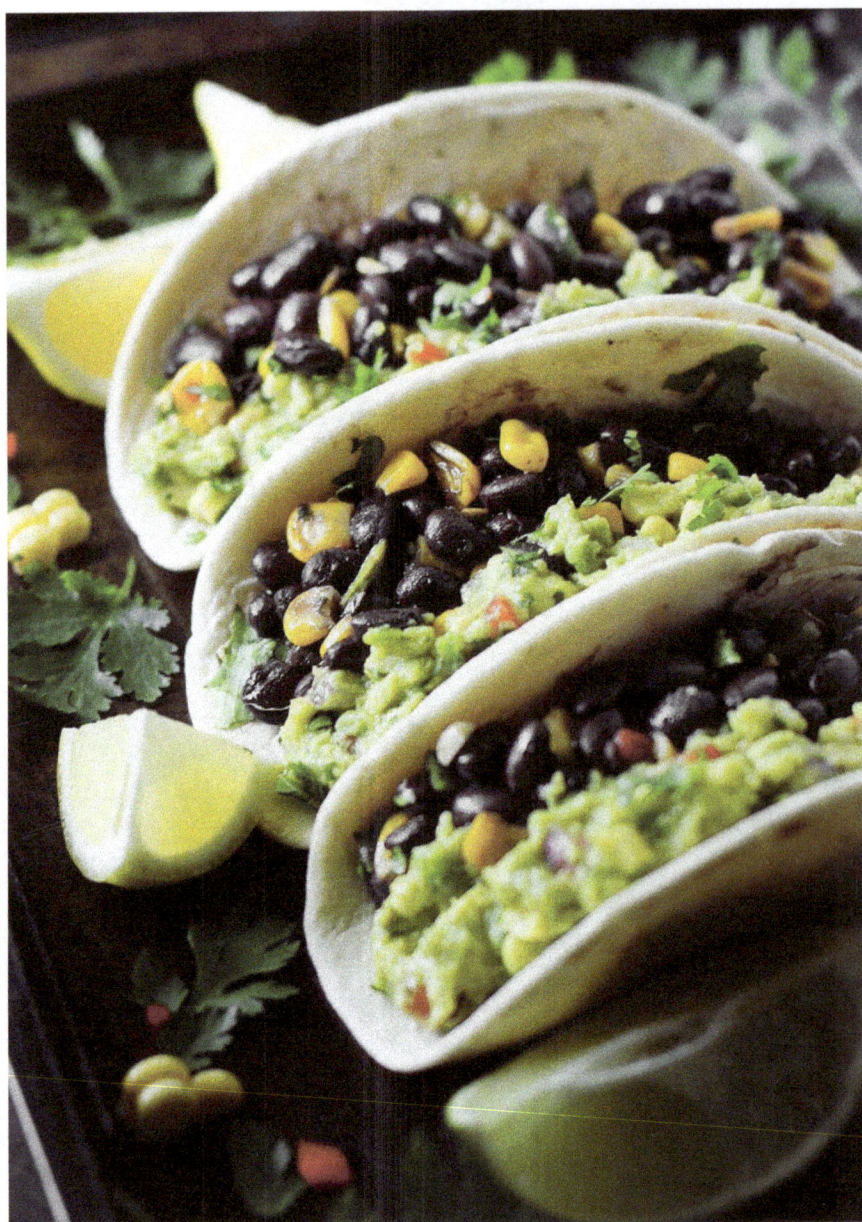

Table of contents

Grilled Turnip and Beetroots

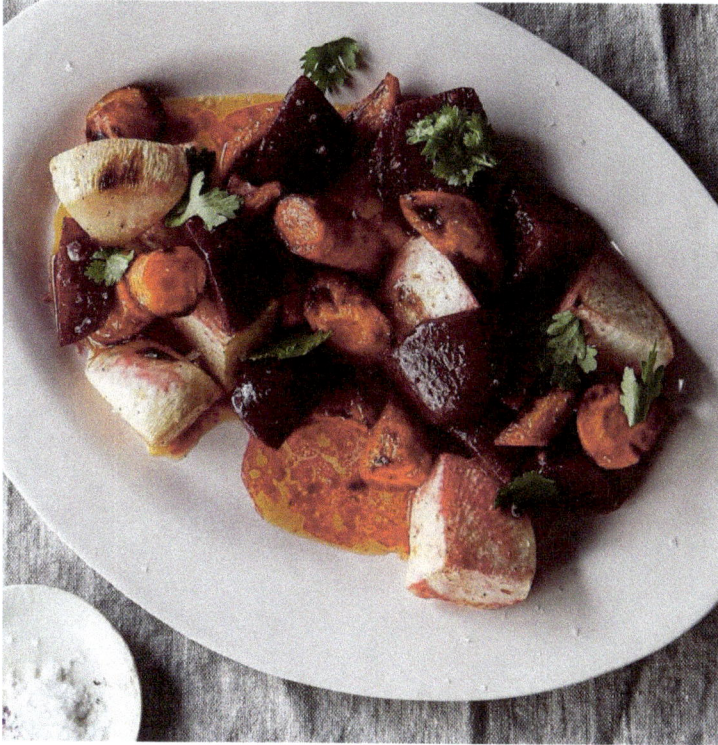

Ingredients

- 1 large turnip, peeled and cut lengthwise

- 1 large carrot, peeled and cut lengthwise

- 1 medium Beetroot , peeled and cut in half lengthwise

Dressing Ingredients

- 6 tbsp. sesame oil

- Sea salt, to taste

- 3 tbsp. distilled white vinegar

- 1 tsp. Egg-free mayonnaise

Directions:

Marinate the vegetable with the dressing or marinade ingredients for 15 to 30 min. Grill for 4 minutes over medium heat or until the vegetable becomes tender.

Grilled Water Chestnuts and Mangoes

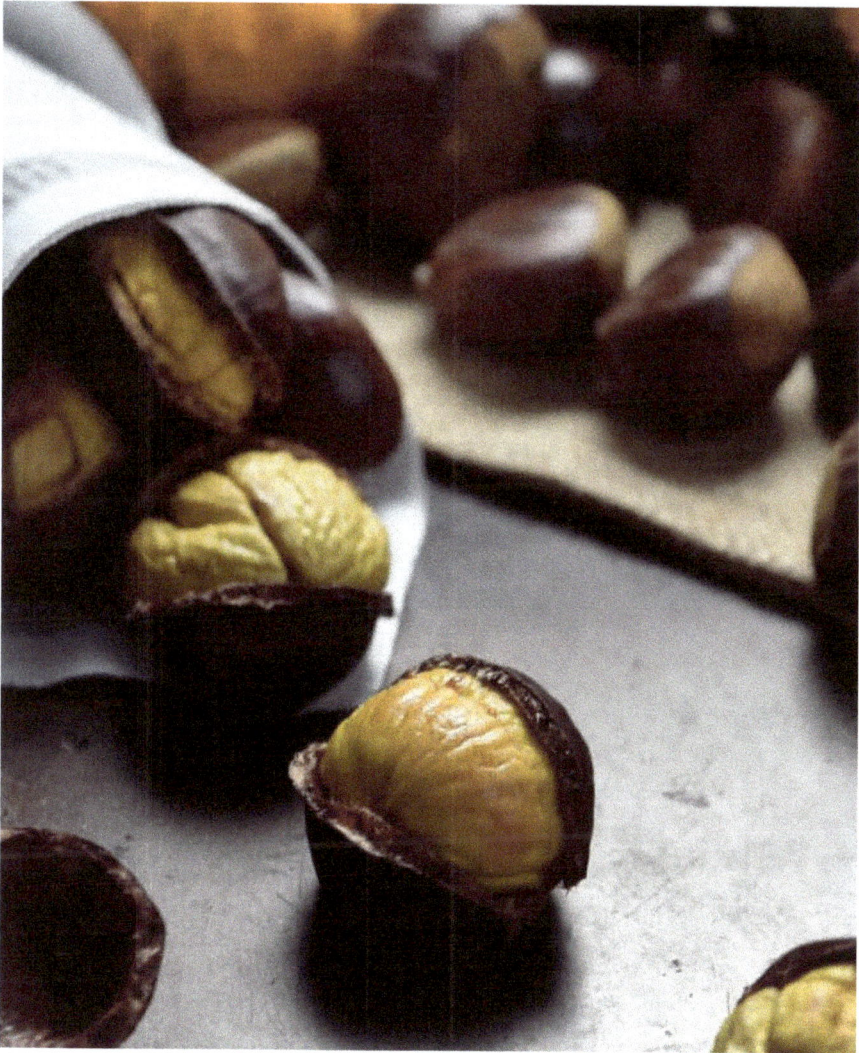

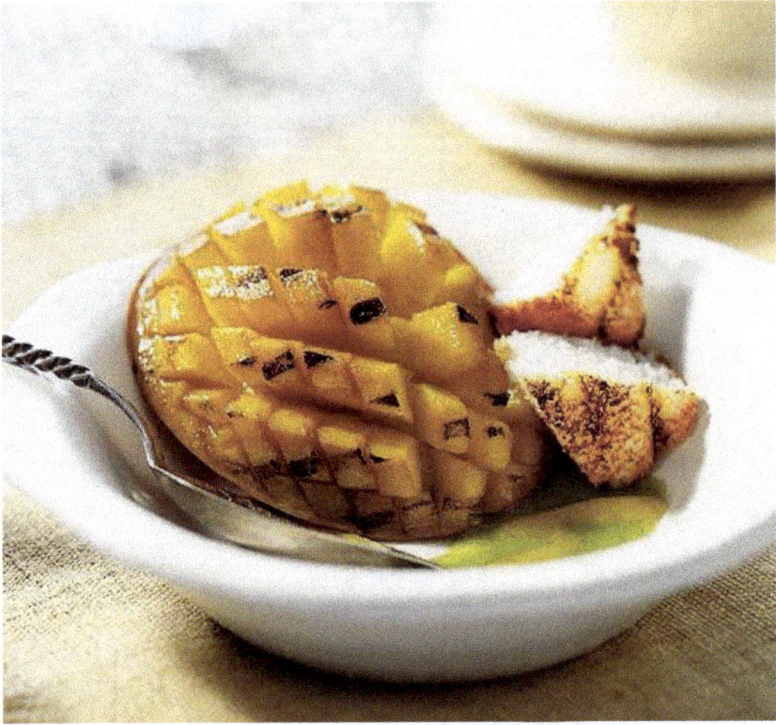

Ingredients

- 1/2 cup water chestnuts

- 2 large mangoes, cut lengthwise and pitted

<u>Dressing Ingredients</u>

- 6 tbsp. sesame oil

- Sea salt, to taste

- 3 tbsp. distilled white vinegar

- 1 tsp. Egg-free mayonnaise

Directions:

Marinate the vegetable with the dressing or marinade ingredients for 15 to 30 min. Grill for 4 minutes over medium heat or until the vegetable becomes tender. For the mango, grill only until you start seeing brown grill marks.

Grilled Artichoke Hearts and Water Chestnuts

Ingredients

- ½ cup canned artichoke hearts
- 1/2 cup water chestnuts
- 10 pcs. Brussel Sprouts

Dressing Ingredients

- 6 tbsp. olive oil
- Sea salt, to taste
- 3 tbsp. white wine vinegar
- 1 tsp. Egg-free mayonnaise

Directions:

Marinate the vegetable with the dressing or marinade ingredients for 15 to 30 min. Grill for 4 minutes over medium heat or until the vegetable becomes tender.

Grilled Assorted Bell Peppers with Broccolini Florets Recipe

Ingredients

- 1 Green Bell Pepper, cut in half
- 2 beetroots, peeled and sliced lengthwise
- 1 red Bell Pepper, cut in half
- 10 Broccolini Florets

Marinade Ingredients:

- 6 tbsp. extra virgin olive oil
- Sea salt, to taste
- 3 tbsp. distilled white vinegar
- 1 tsp. Dijon mustard

Directions:

Marinate the vegetable with the dressing or marinade ingredients for 15 to 30 min. Grill for 4 minutes over medium heat or until the vegetable becomes tender.

Grilled Portobello and Rutabaga

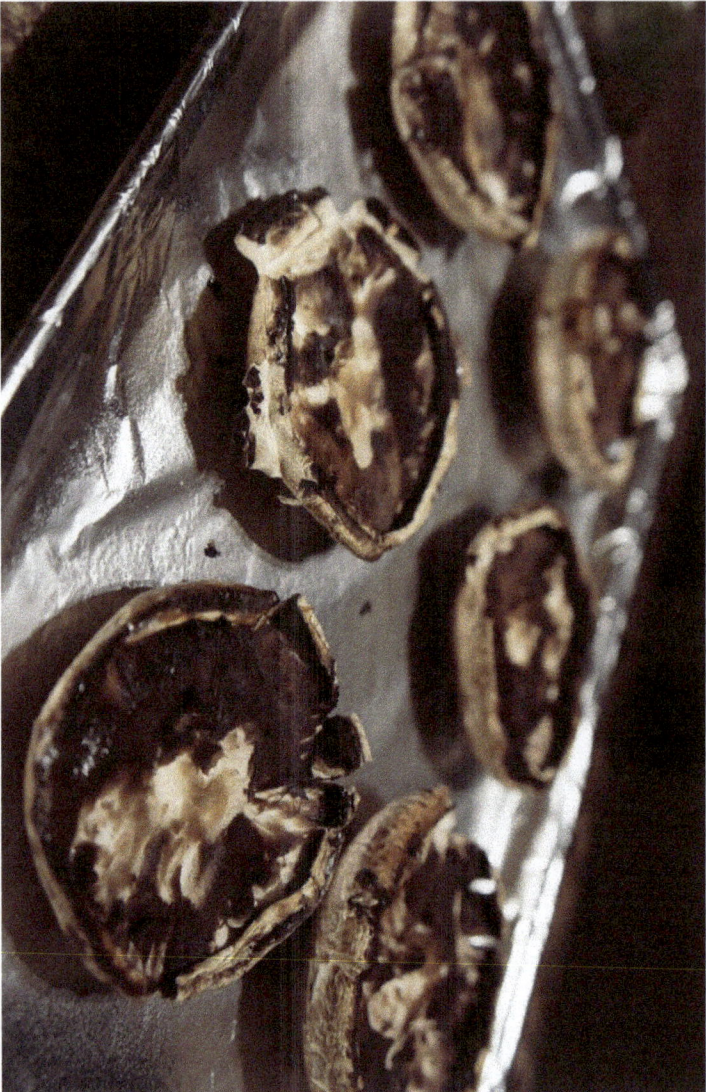

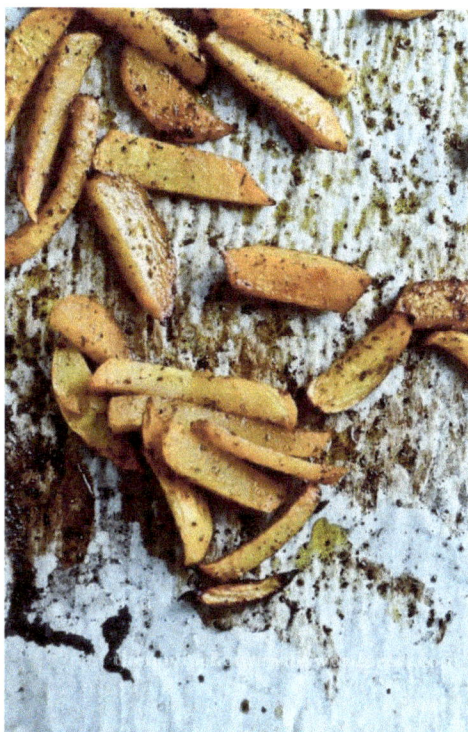

Ingredients

- 1 medium Rutabaga, peeled and cut in half lengthwise

- 5 pcs. Portobello mushrooms, rinsed and drained

- 1 medium red onion, cut into ½ inch rings but don't separate into individual rings

Dressing Ingredients

- 6 tbsp. extra virgin olive oil

- Sea salt, to taste

- 3 tbsp. Balsamic vinegar

- 1 tsp. Dijon mustard

Directions:

Marinate the vegetable with the dressing or marinade ingredients for 15 to 30 min. Grill for 4 minutes over medium heat or until the vegetable becomes tender.

Grilled Brussel Sprouts Cauliflower and Rutabaga

Ingredients

- 1 medium Rutabaga, peeled and cut in half lengthwise
- 10 Cauliflower florets
- 5 pcs. Brussel Sprouts
- 1 bunch of collard greens

Dressing Ingredients

- 6 tbsp. olive oil
- Sea salt, to taste
- 3 tbsp. white wine vinegar
- 1 tsp. English mustard

Directions:

Marinate the vegetable with the dressing or marinade ingredients for 15 to 30 min. Grill for 4 minutes over medium heat or until the vegetable becomes tender.

Grilled Water Chestnuts Swiss Chard and Asparagus Recipe

Ingredients

- 1/2 cup water chestnuts

- 1 bunch of swiss chard

- 6 pcs. Asparagus

- <u>Dressing Ingredients</u>

- 6 tbsp. extra virgin olive oil

- Sea salt, to taste

- 3 tbsp. apple cider vinegar

- 1 tbsp. honey

- 1 tsp. Egg-free mayonnaise

Directions:

Marinate the vegetable with the dressing or marinade ingredients for 15 to 30 min. Grill for 4 minutes over medium heat or until the vegetable becomes tender.

Grilled Asparagus Pineapple and Green Beans

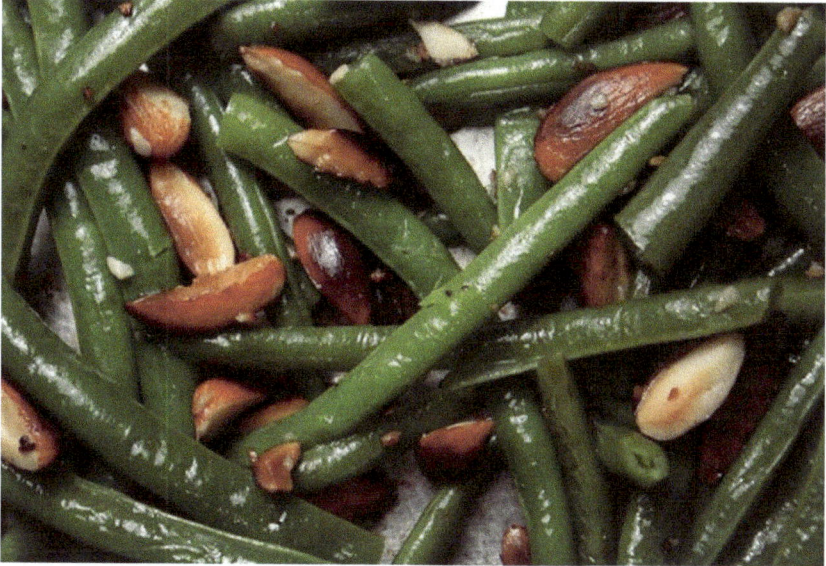

Ingredients

- 1 medium Rutabaga, peeled and cut in half lengthwise

- 10 pcs. Asparagus

- 1 medium Pineapple, cut into 1/2 inch slices

- 1 bunch of collard greens

Dressing Ingredients

- 6 tbsp. sesame oil

- Sea salt, to taste

- 3 tbsp. distilled white vinegar

- 1 tsp. Egg-free mayonnaise

Directions:

Marinate the vegetable with the dressing or marinade ingredients for 15 to 30 min. Grill for 4 minutes over medium heat or until the vegetable becomes tender.

Asparagus Dressing

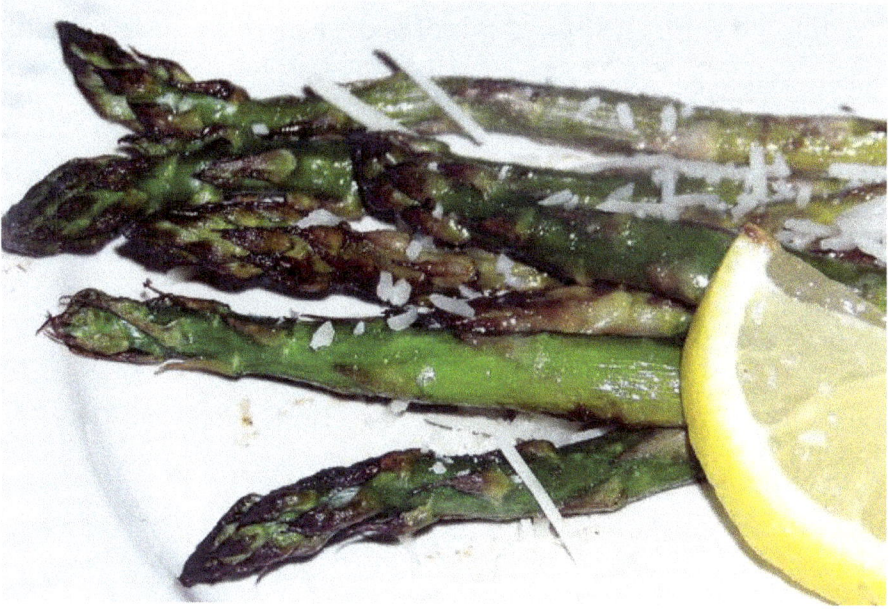

Ingredients

- 6 tbsp. sesame oil

- Sea salt, to taste

- 3 tbsp. distilled white vinegar

- 1 tsp. Egg-free mayonnaise

Directions:

Marinate the vegetable with the dressing or marinade ingredients for 15 to 30 min. Grill for 4 minutes over medium heat or until the vegetable becomes tender.

Grilled Broccoli & Swiss Chard

Ingredients

- 2 green Bell Peppers, cut in half
- 1 bunch of swiss chard
- 5 Broccoli Florets Dressing Ingredients
- 6 tbsp. sesame oil
- Sea salt, to taste
- 3 tbsp. distilled white vinegar
- 1 tsp. Egg-free mayonnaise

Directions:

Marinate the vegetable with the dressing or marinade ingredients for 15 to 30 min. Grill for 4 minutes over medium heat or until the vegetable becomes tender.

Grilled Water Chestnuts and Green Beans

Ingredients

- 10 Broccolini Florets

- 10 pcs. Asparagus

- 1/2 cup water chestnuts

- 10 Green Beans

- <u>Marinade Ingredients:</u>

- 6 tbsp. extra virgin olive oil

- Sea salt, to taste

- 3 tbsp. distilled white vinegar

- 1 tsp. Dijon mustard

Directions:

Marinate the vegetable with the dressing or marinade ingredients for 15 to 30 min. Grill for 4 minutes over medium heat or until the vegetable becomes tender.

Grilled Turnip Greens and Okra

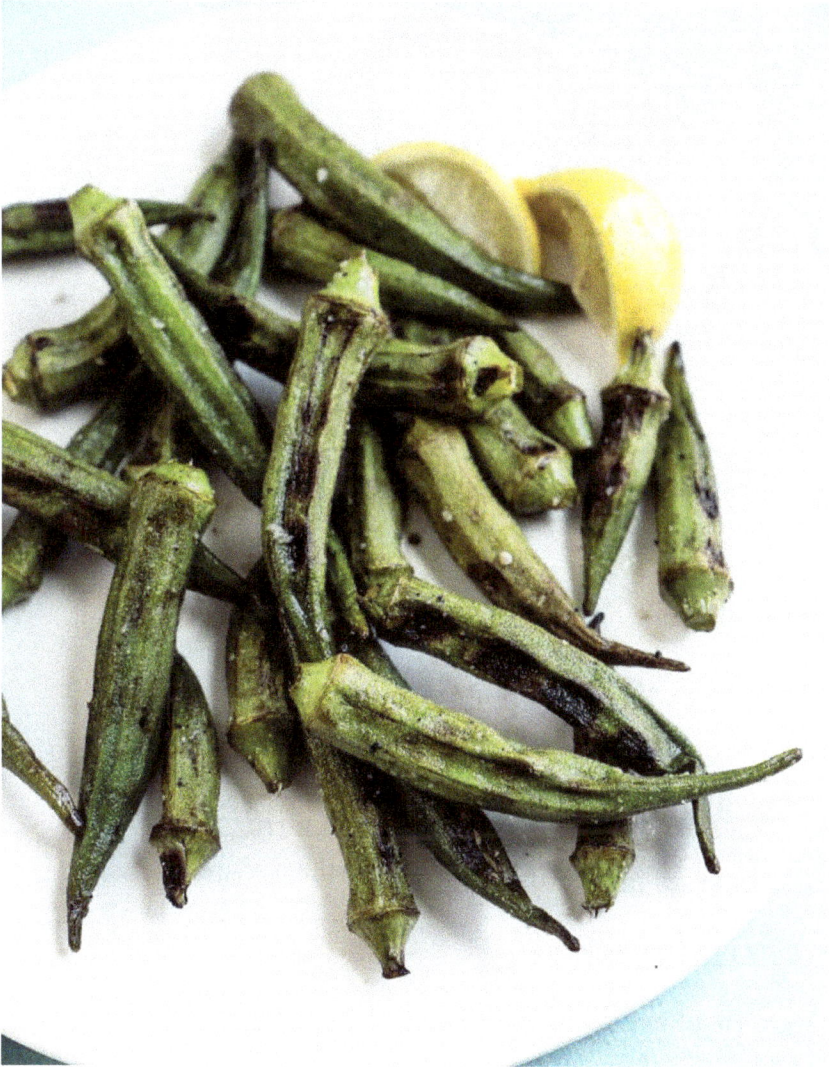

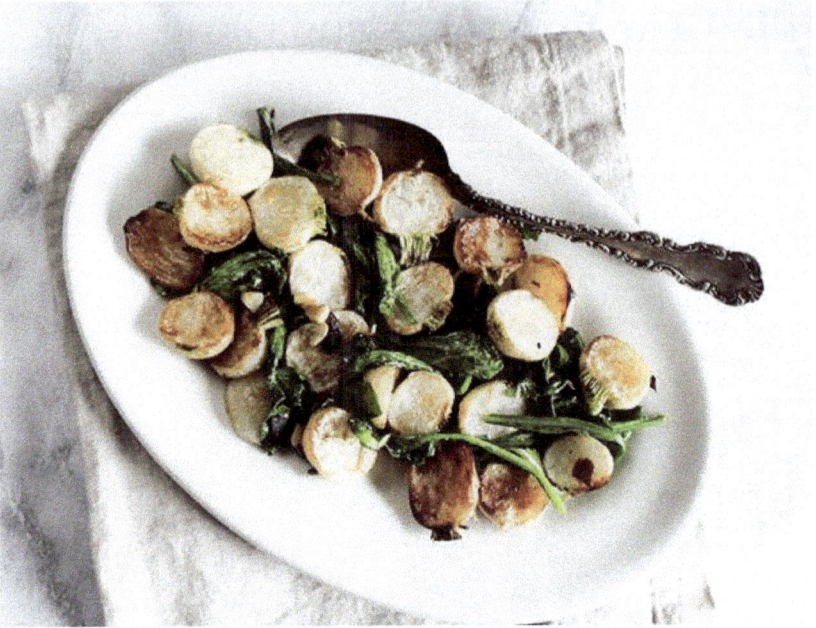

Ingredients

- 5 pcs. Okra

- 1 bunch of turnip greens

- 2 large red onions, cut into ½ inch rings but don't separate into individual rings

Dressing Ingredients

- 6 tbsp. extra virgin olive oil

- Sea salt, to taste

- 3 tbsp. Balsamic vinegar

- 1 tsp. Dijon mustard

Directions:

Marinate the vegetable with the dressing or marinade ingredients for 15 to 30 min. Grill for 4 minutes over medium heat or until the vegetable becomes tender.

Grilled Beetroots and Purple Cabbage

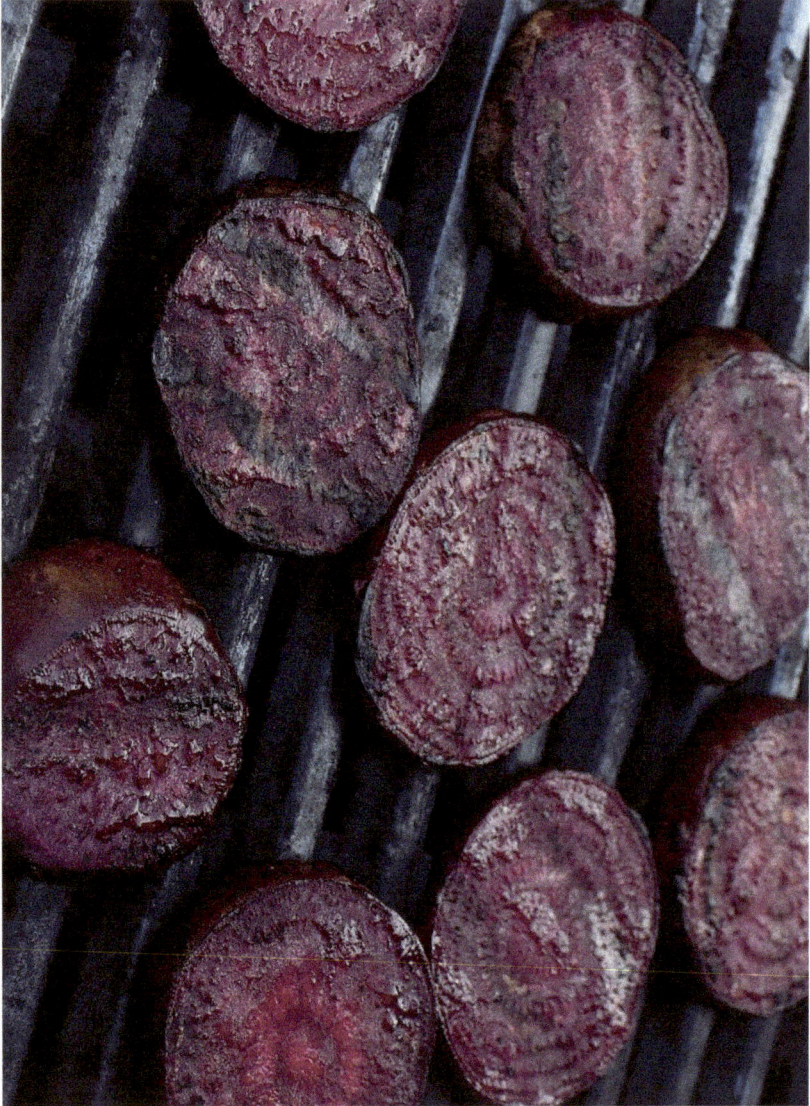

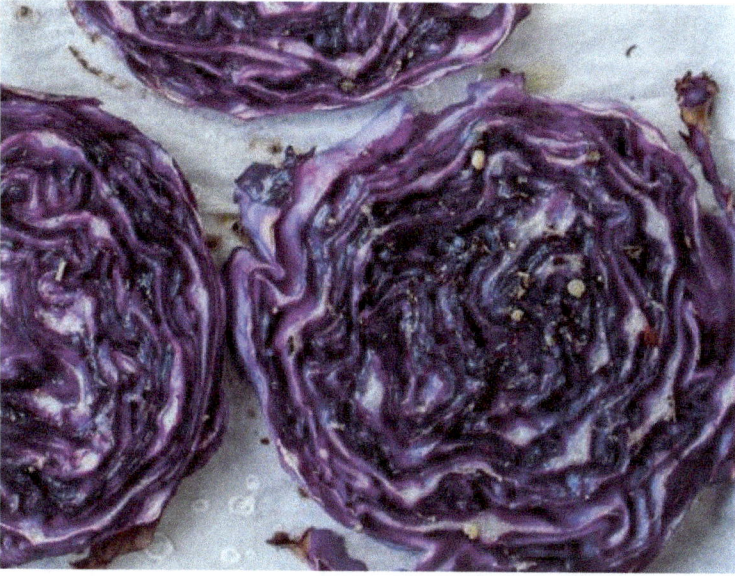

Ingredients

- 1 large Parsnip, cut lengthwise

- 1 Purple cabbage

- 2 beetroots, peeled and sliced lengthwise

- 2 large Zucchinis, cut lengthwise and cut in half

Dressing Ingredients

- 6 tbsp. olive oil

- Sea salt, to taste

- 3 tbsp. white wine vinegar

- 1 tsp. English mustard

Directions:

Marinate the vegetable with the dressing or marinade ingredients for 15 to 30 min. Grill for 4 minutes over medium heat or until the vegetable becomes tender.

Grilled Turnip and Endives

Ingredients

- 1 large Turnip, cut lengthwise
- 2 green Bell Peppers, cut in half
- 1 bunch of endives
- Dressing Ingredients
- 6 tbsp. extra virgin olive oil
- Sea salt, to taste
- 3 tbsp. apple cider vinegar
- 1 tbsp. honey
- 1 tsp. Egg-free mayonnaise

Directions:

Marinate the vegetable with the dressing or marinade ingredients for 15 to 30 min. Grill for 4 minutes over medium heat or until the vegetable becomes tender.

Grilled Green Beans and Pineapple

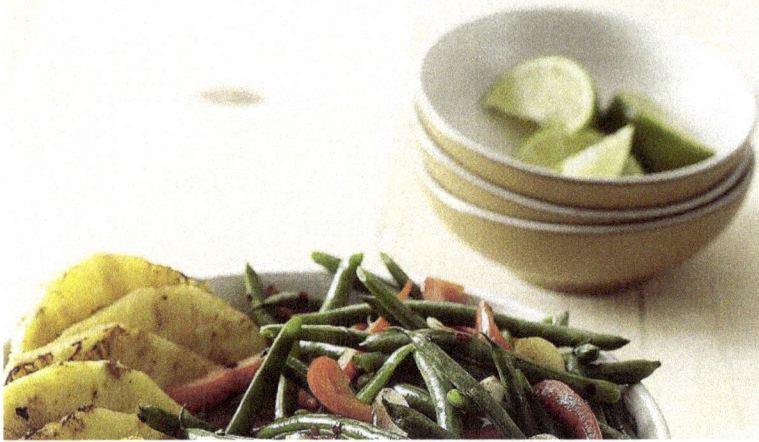

Ingredients

- 1 large Turnip, cut lengthwise

- 1 medium Pineapple, cut into 1/2 inch slices

- 10 Green Beans

Dressing Ingredients

- 6 tbsp. sesame oil

- Sea salt, to taste

- 3 tbsp. distilled white vinegar

- 1 tsp. Egg-free mayonnaise

Directions:

Marinate the vegetable with the dressing or marinade ingredients for 15 to 30 min. Grill for 4 minutes over medium heat or until the vegetable becomes tender.

Grilled Turnip and Zucchini

Ingredients

- 1 large Turnip, cut lengthwise
- 1 bunch of turnip greens
- 1 large zucchini , cut lengthwise into ½ inch slabs
- 2 small red onions, cut into ½ inch rings but don't separate into individual rings

<u>Dressing Ingredients</u>

- 6 tbsp. extra virgin olive oil
- Sea salt, to taste
- 3 tbsp. Balsamic vinegar
- 1 tsp. Dijon mustard

Directions:

Marinate the vegetable with the dressing or marinade ingredients for 15 to 30 min. Grill for 4 minutes over medium heat or until the vegetable becomes tender.

Grilled Portobello Mushrooms and Broccolini Florets

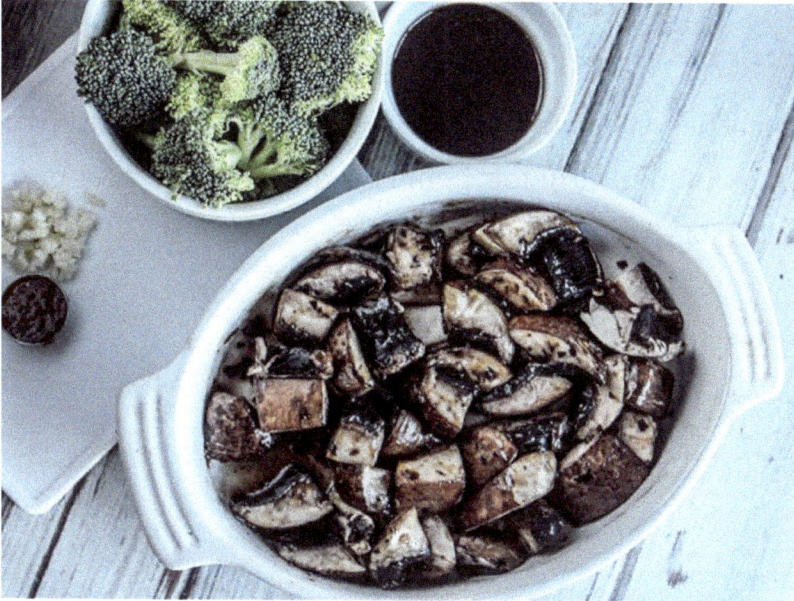

Ingredients

- 10 Broccolini Florets

- 10 pcs. Asparagus Corns, cut lengthwise

- 5 pcs. Portobello mushrooms, rinsed and drained

Marinade Ingredients:

- 6 tbsp. extra virgin olive oil

- Sea salt, to taste

- 3 tbsp. distilled white vinegar

- 1 tsp. Dijon mustard

Directions:

Marinate the vegetable with the dressing or marinade ingredients for 15 to 30 min. Grill for 4 minutes over medium heat or until the vegetable becomes tender.

Grilled Beetroots and Artichoke Hearts

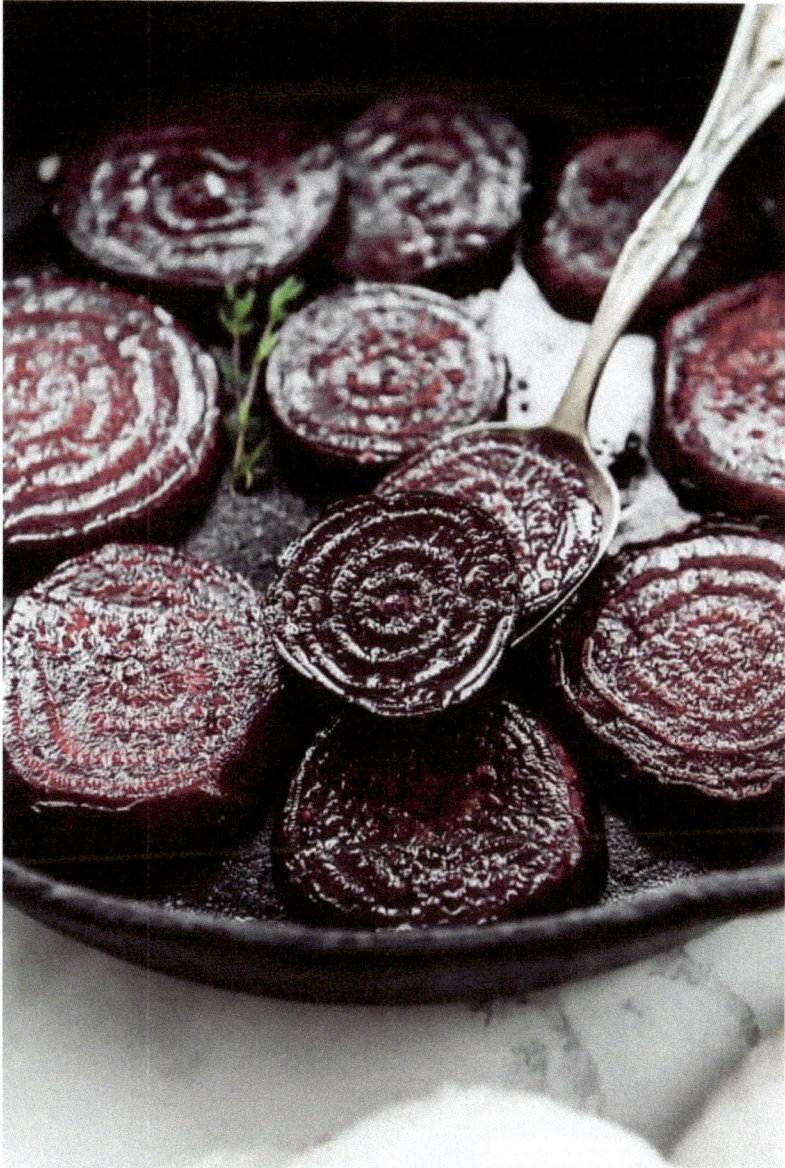

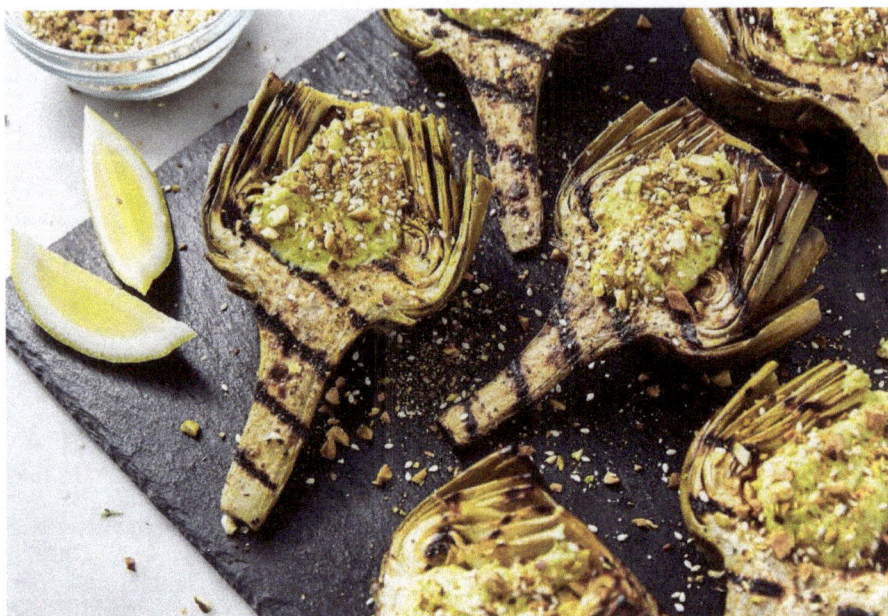

Ingredients

- ½ cup canned artichoke hearts

- 10 Broccolini Florets

- 2 beetroots, peeled and sliced lengthwise

Dressing Ingredients

- 6 tbsp. sesame oil

- Sea salt, to taste

- 3 tbsp. distilled white vinegar

- 1 tsp. Egg-free mayonnaise

Directions:

Marinate the vegetable with the dressing or marinade ingredients for 15 to 30 min. Grill for 4 minutes over medium heat or until the vegetable becomes tender.

Grilled Baby Carrots and Zucchini

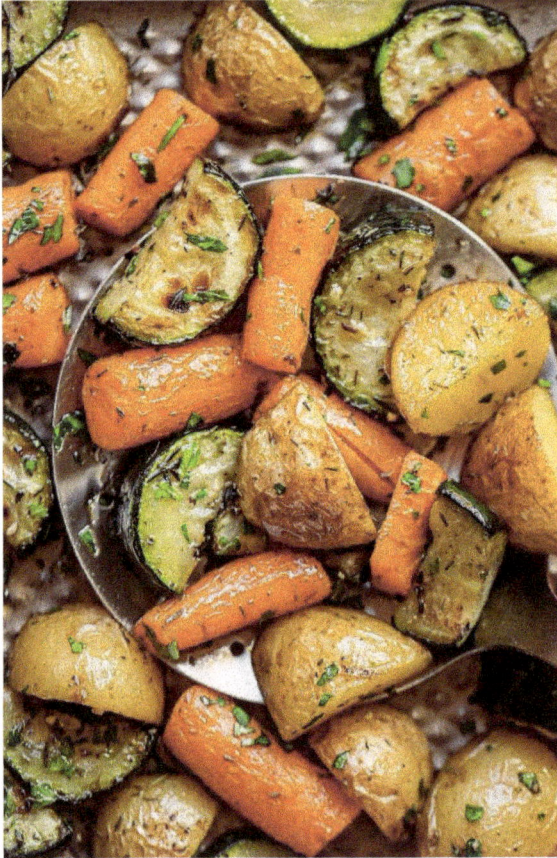

Ingredients

- 7 pcs. baby carrots

- 2 large zucchini, cut lengthwise into ½ inch slabs

- 2 large red onions, cut into ½ inch rings but don't separate into individual rings

Dressing Ingredients

- 6 tbsp. olive oil

- Sea salt, to taste

- 3 tbsp. white wine vinegar

- 1 tsp. Egg-free mayonnaise

Directions:

Marinate the vegetable with the dressing or marinade ingredients for 15 to 30 min. Grill for 4 minutes over medium heat or until the vegetable becomes tender.

Grilled Water Chestnuts Baby Carrots and Artichoke Hearts

Ingredients

- 1 cup canned artichoke hearts
- 1/2 cup canned water chestnuts
- 8 pcs. baby carrots

Dressing Ingredients

- 6 tbsp. olive oil
- Sea salt, to taste
- 3 bsp. white wine vinegar
- 1 tsp. English mustard

Directions:

Marinate the vegetable with the dressing or marinade ingredients for 15 to 30 min. Grill for 4 minutes over medium heat or until the vegetable becomes tender.

Grilled Rutabaga Zucchini and Onions

Ingredients

- 1 medium Rutabaga, peeled and cut in half lengthwise
- 2 large zucchini , cut lengthwise into ½ inch slabs
- 2 large red onions, cut into ½ inch rings but don't separate into individual rings

Dressing Ingredients

- 6 tbsp. olive oil
- Sea salt, to taste
- 3 tbsp. white wine vinegar
- 1 tsp. Egg-free mayonnaise

Directions:

Marinate the vegetable with the dressing or marinade ingredients for 15 to 30 min. Grill for 4 minutes over medium heat or until the vegetable becomes tender.

Grilled Rutabaga Broccolini Florets and Bell Peppers

Ingredients

- 1 medium Rutabaga, peeled and cut in half lengthwise

- 2 green Bell Peppers, cut in half

- 10 Broccolini Florets

<u>Dressing Ingredients</u>

- 6 tbsp. sesame oil

- Sea salt, to taste

- 3 tbsp. distilled white vinegar

- 1 tsp. Egg-free mayonnaise

Directions:

Marinate the vegetable with the dressing or marinade ingredients for 15 to 30 min. Grill for 4 minutes over medium heat or until the vegetable becomes tender.

Grilled Baby Carrots and Winter Squash

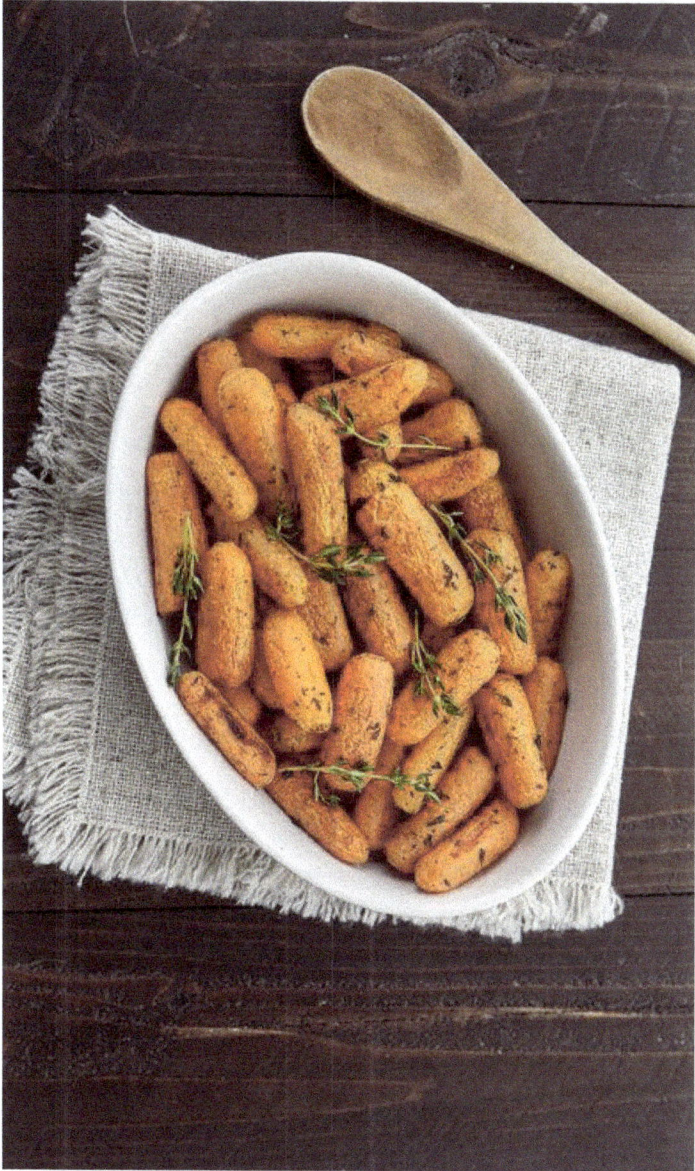

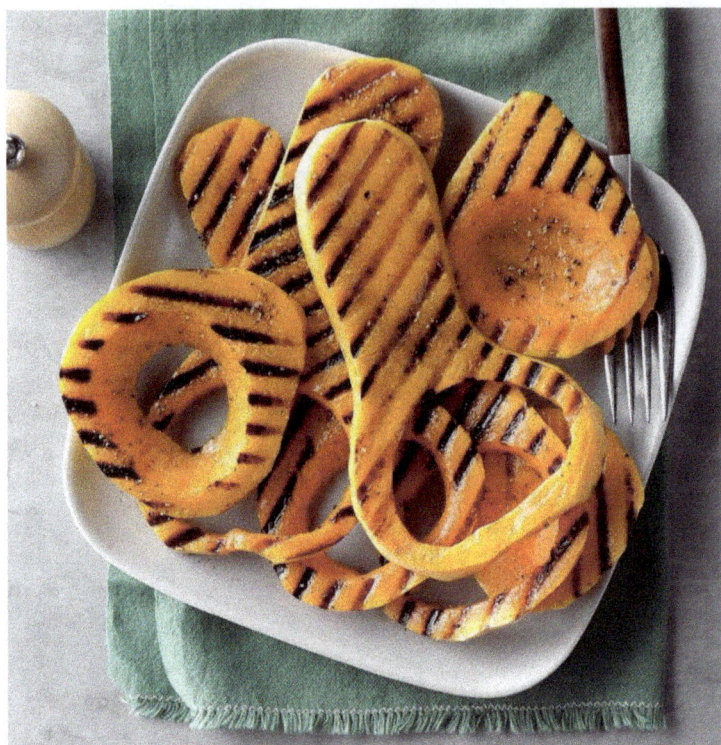

Ingredients

- 1 winter squash, peeled and sliced lengthwise

- ½ cup baby carrots

- 1 bunch of turnip greens

- 2 large red onions, cut into ½ inch rings but don't separate into individual rings

<u>Dressing Ingredients</u>

- 6 tbsp. extra virgin olive oil

- Sea salt, to taste

- 3 tbsp. Balsamic vinegar

- 1 tsp. Dijon mustard

Directions:

Marinate the vegetable with the dressing or marinade ingredients for 15 to 30 min. Grill for 4 minutes over medium heat or until the vegetable becomes tender

Grilled Beetroots and Artichoke Hearts in Viniagrette

Ingredients

- 1 cup canned artichoke hearts

- 2 beetroots, peeled and sliced lengthwise

Dressing Ingredients

- 6 tbsp. olive oil

- Sea salt, to taste

- 3 tbsp. white wine vinegar

- 1 tsp. English mustard

Directions:

Marinate the vegetable with the dressing or marinade ingredients for 15 to 30 min. Grill for 4 minutes over medium heat or until the vegetable becomes tender.

Grilled Beetroots Artichoke Hearts and Asparagus

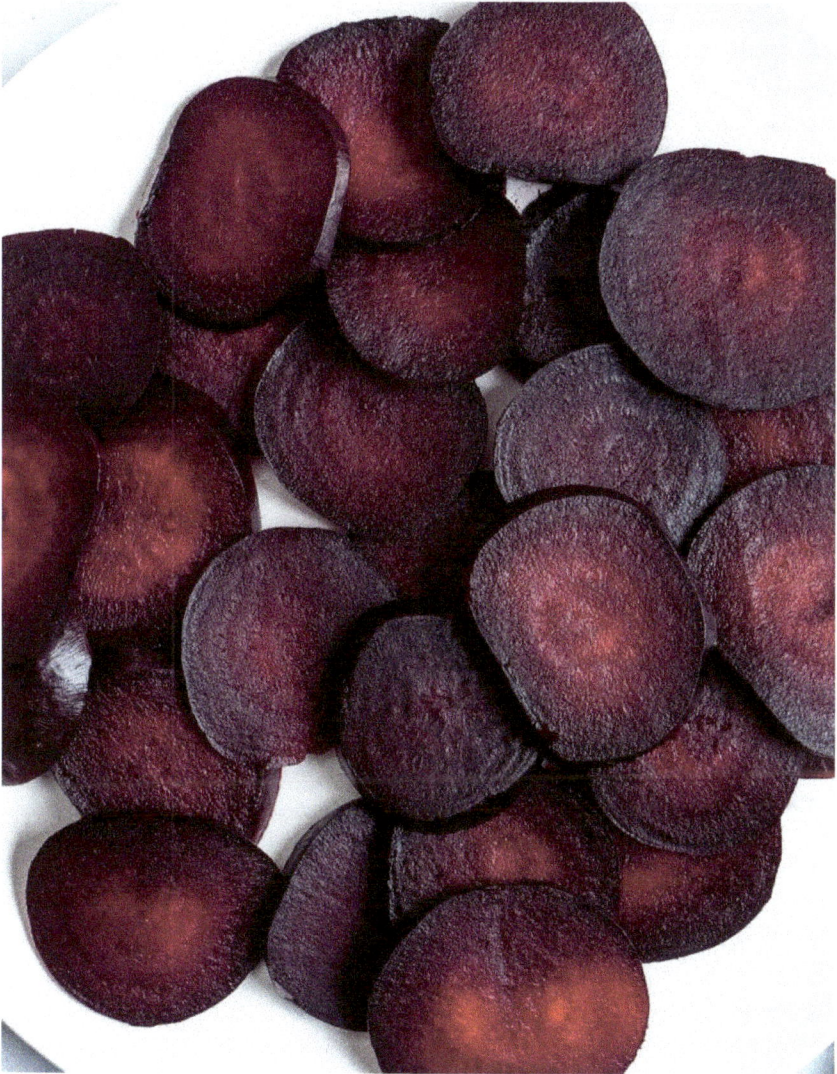

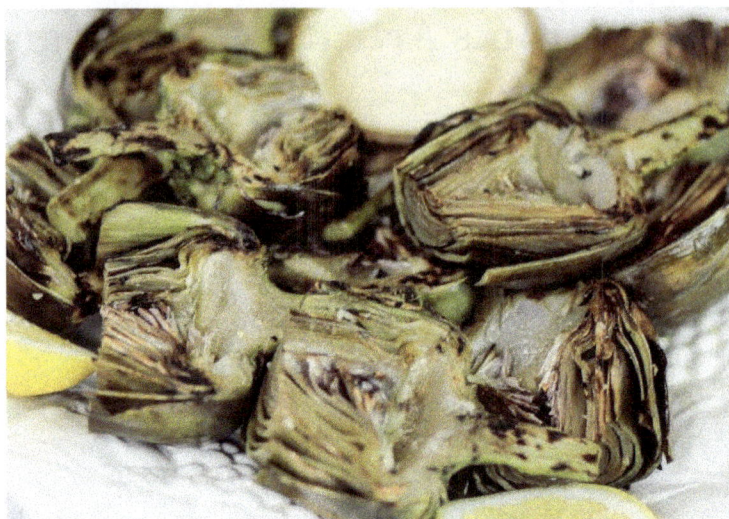

Ingredients

- ½ cup canned artichoke hearts

- 2 beetroots, peeled and sliced lengthwise

- 10 pcs. Asparagus

<u>Dressing Ingredients</u>

- 6 tbsp. extra virgin olive oil

- Sea salt, to taste

- 3 tbsp. apple cider vinegar

- 1 tbsp. honey

- 1 tsp. Egg-free mayonnaise

Directions:

Marinate the vegetable with the dressing or marinade ingredients for 15 to 30 min. Grill for 4 minutes over medium heat or until the vegetable becomes tender.

Grilled Summer Squash with Balsamic Glaze

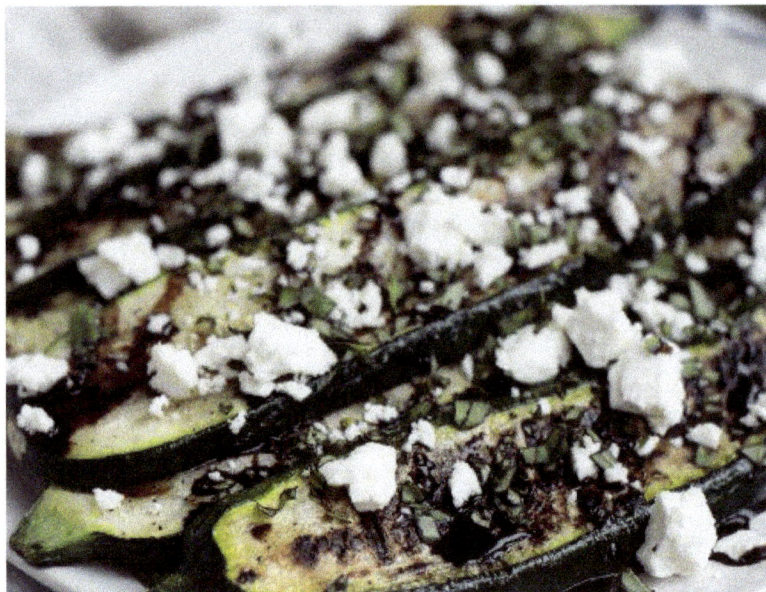

Ingredients

- 1 summer squash, peeled and sliced lengthwise

Dressing Ingredients

- 6 tbsp. extra virgin olive oil

- Sea salt, to taste

- 3 tbsp. Balsamic vinegar

- 1 tsp. Dijon mustard

Directions:

Marinate the vegetable with the dressing or marinade ingredients for 15 to 30 min. Grill for 4 minutes over medium heat or until the vegetable becomes tender.

Kidney Beans & Button Mushrooms with Pesto Sauce

Ingredients

- 2 red onions
- 7 garlic cloves
- 1 ancho chili, minced
- 1 tbsp. lime juice
- 4 cups vegetable broth
- 1 can water (I use the can of diced tomatoes to grab all the leftover flavor)
- 8 oz. dried kidney beans
- 1 15 oz can button mushrooms
- 3 tablespoons pesto sauce
- 1 teaspoons dried basil, coarsely chopped
- 1 tsp. dried Italian seasoning
- 1/2 cup uncooked rice
- 1/4 teaspoon sea salt

Directions:

Put all of the ingredients into slow cooker. Cook on low for 8 hours or high for 4 hours. Serve with toppings such as shredded vegan cheese, avocado, green onion and cilantro

Slow Cooked Quinoa and Tomatoes

Ingredients

- 1 red onion, chopped 1 white onion, chopped

- 8 garlic cloves, minced

- 1 tsp. shallot, minced

- 1 15 oz can diced tomatoes

- 4 cups vegetable broth

- 1 can water (I use the can of diced tomatoes to grab all the leftover flavor)

- 2 15 oz cans sliced porcini mushrooms

- 2 tablespoons chili powder

- 2 teaspoons cumin
  1 tablespoon oregano

- 1/2 cup uncooked quinoa

- 1/4 teaspoon sea salt

Directions:

Put all of the ingredients into slow cooker. Cook on low for 8 hours or high for 4 hours. Serve with toppings such as shredded vegan cheese, avocado, green onion and cilantro

Black Rice with Enoki Mushroom in Chimichurri

Ingredients

- 2 red onions

- 7 garlic cloves

- 1 ancho chili, minced

- 1 tbsp. lime juice

- 1 15 oz can diced tomatoes

- 4 cups vegetable broth
  1 can water (I use the can of diced tomatoes to grab all the leftover flavor)

- 1 8 oz can enoki mushrooms

- 2 tablespoons garlic, minced

- 2 teaspoons chili powder

- 1 tablespoon chimichurri

- 1/2 cup uncooked black rice

- 1/4 teaspoon sea salt

Directions:

Put all of the ingredients into slow cooker. Cook on low for 8 hours or high for 4 hours. Serve with toppings such as shredded vegan cheese, avocado, green onion and cilantro

Quinoa and Enoki Mushrooms

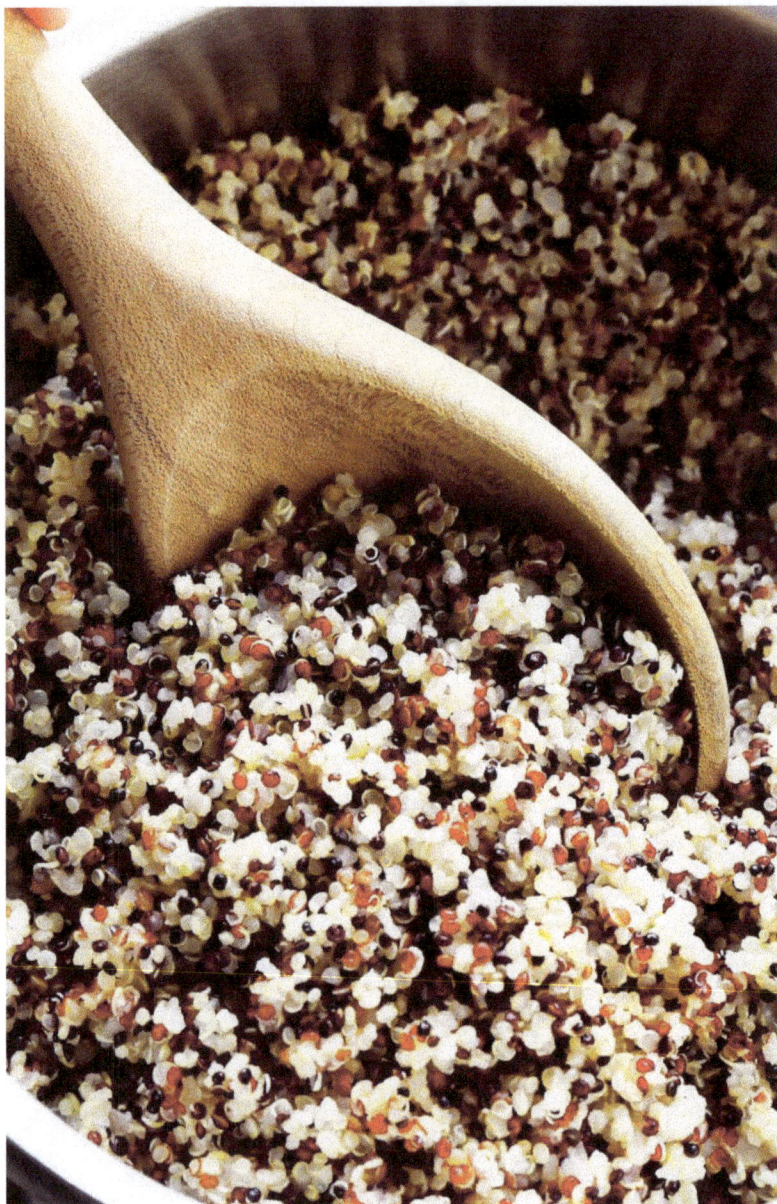

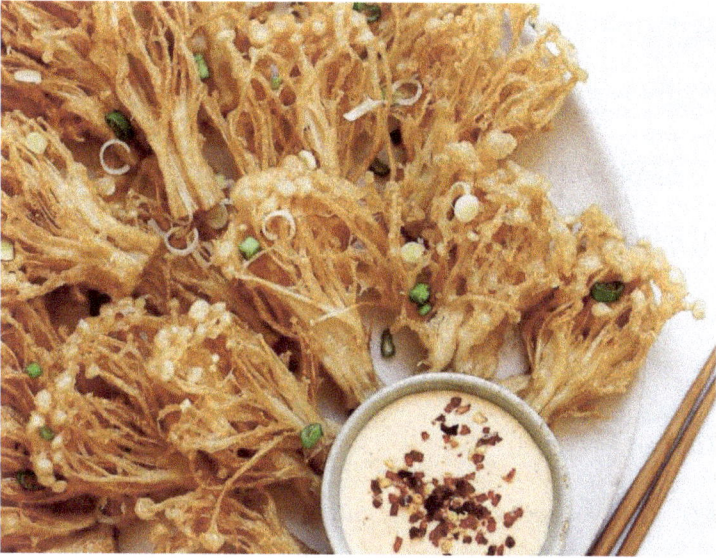

Ingredients

- 2 red onion, chopped

- 7 garlic cloves, minced

- 8 jalapeno peppers, minced

- 1 tbsp. lemon juice

- 4 cups vegetable broth

- 1 can water (I use the can of diced tomatoes to grab all the leftover flavor)

- 1 15 oz can enoki mushrooms

- 1 15 oz can button mushrooms

- 2 tablespoons chili powder

61

- 2 teaspoons cumin

- 1 tablespoon oregano

- 1/2 cup uncooked quinoa

- 1/4 teaspoon sea salt

Directions:

Put all of the ingredients into slow cooker. Cook on low for 8 hours or high for 4 hours. Serve with toppings such as shredded vegan cheese, avocado, green onion and cilantro

Brown Rice with Vegan Chorizo and Ancho Chili

Ingredients

- 2 red onions

- 7 garlic cloves

- 1 ancho chili, minced

- 1 tbsp. lime juice

- 4 cups vegetable broth

- 1 can water (I use the can of diced tomatoes to grab all the leftover flavor)

- 1 cup crimini mushrooms

- 1/2 cup vegan Chorizo (Soyrizo), crumbled

- 2 tablespoons annatto seeds

- 2 teaspoons cumin

- 1 tsp. cayenne pepper

- 1/2 cup uncooked brown rice

- 1/4 teaspoon sea salt

Directions:

Put all of the ingredients into slow cooker. Cook on low for 8 hours or high for 4 hours. Serve with toppings such as shredded vegan cheese, avocado, green onion and cilantro

Split Pea Celery and Leek Soup

Ingredients

- 1 16- oz package

- 1 lb dried green split peas, rinsed

- 1 large leek light green and white portion only, chopped and thoroughly cleaned

- 3 celery ribs diced

- 2 large carrots diced

- 4 garlic clove minced

- 1/4 cup chopped fresh parsley

- 6 cups vegetable broth

- 1/2 t ground black pepper

- 1 tsp sea salt or to taste

- 1 bay leaf

Directions:

Pour all of the ingredients in a slow cooker and combine thoroughly. Cover a cook on low heat for 7 and a half hours or high 3 and a half hours. Take out the bay leaf.

Slow Cooked Chick Peas and Vegetarian Sausage

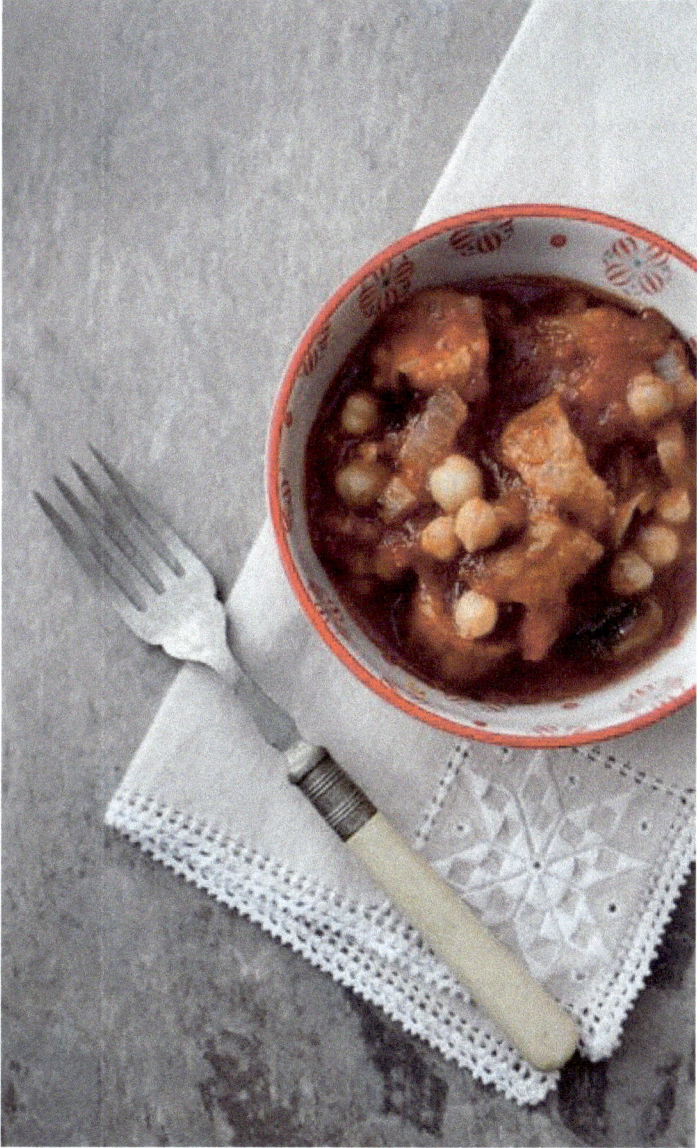

Ingredients

- 2 teaspoons extra virgin olive oil
- 1 medium red onion, diced (about 2 cups)
- 4 medium cloves garlic, minced (about 2 teaspoons)
- 2 teaspoons ground coriander
- 2 teaspoons ground cumin
- 1/2 teaspoon garam masala
- 1/2 teaspoon ground ginger
- 1/4 teaspoon turmeric
- 1/4 teaspoon crushed red pepper flakes
- 1 teaspoon sea salt
- 1 (15-ounce) can diced tomatoes
- 2 tablespoons tomato paste
- 1 cup vegetable stock
- 2 (15-ounce) cans chickpeas, drained and rinsed
- 1/2 cup vegetarian grain meat sausages, crumble
- 1 pound red potatoes, cut into 1/2-inch dice
- 1 lime
- Small bunch fresh cilantro

Equipment:

- 3-quart or larger slow cooker

Directions:

Heat the olive oil in a large pan over medium heat. Sauté the onion until softened and translucent. This takes about 5 minutes. Add in the garlic, coriander, cumin, garam masala, ground ginger, turmeric, red pepper flakes, and sea salt. Cook and stir for 1 minute. Add in the diced tomatoes, tomato paste, and vegetable broth. Combine and pour into the slow cooker. Add the chickpeas and potatoes. Cook on high heat for 4 1/2 hours or low for 9 hours, or until the potatoes become fork-tender. Serve in bowls and garnished with fresh cilantro and lime wedges

Red Potato and Baby Spinach Soup

Ingredients

- 5 cups low sodium vegetable stock

- 3 large red potatoes peeled and chopped

- 1 cup onion chopped

- 2 stalks celery chopped

- 4 cloves garlic crushed

- 1 cup heavy cream

- 1 tsp. dried tarragon

- 2 cups baby spinach

- 6-8 tbsp. sliced almonds

- sea salt and ground black pepper to taste

Directions:

Combine stock, sweet potatoes, onion, celery, and garlic to a 4-quart slow cooker. Cook on low heat for 8 hours or until potatoes become soft. Add almond milk, tarragon, salt and pepper. Blend this mixture for 1-2 minutes with an immersion blender until soup is smooth. Add baby spinach & cover. Let it rest for 20 minutes or until spinach becomes soft. Garnish with almonds and season with sea salt and pepper.

Grilled Zucchinis and Crimini Mushrooms

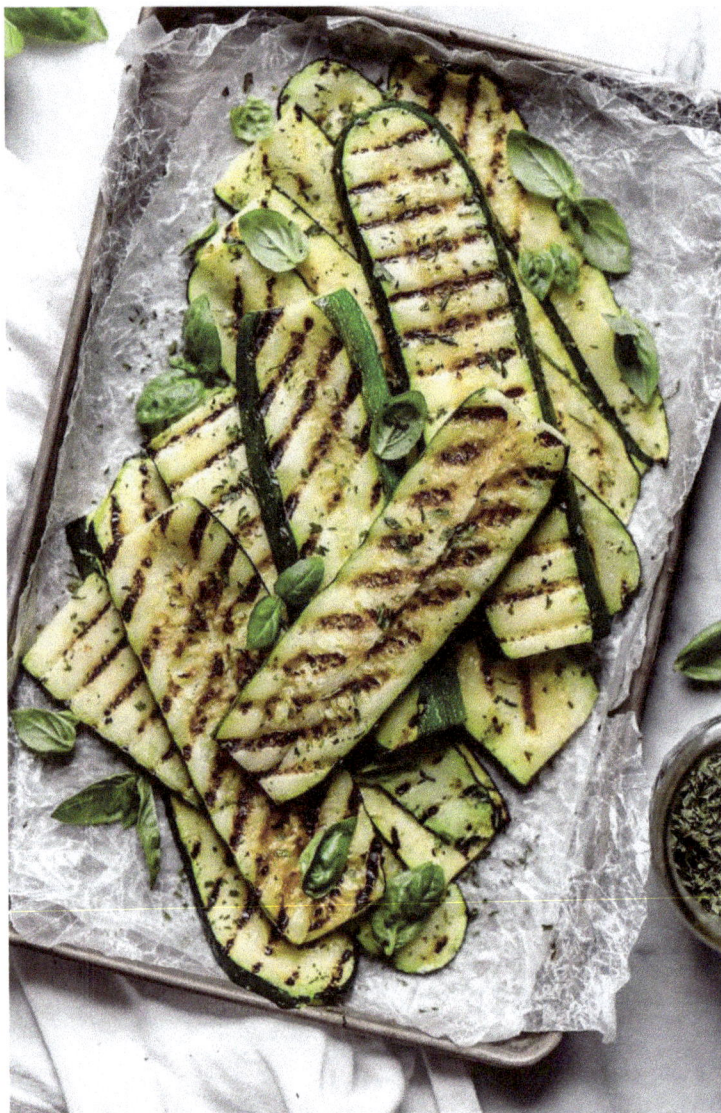

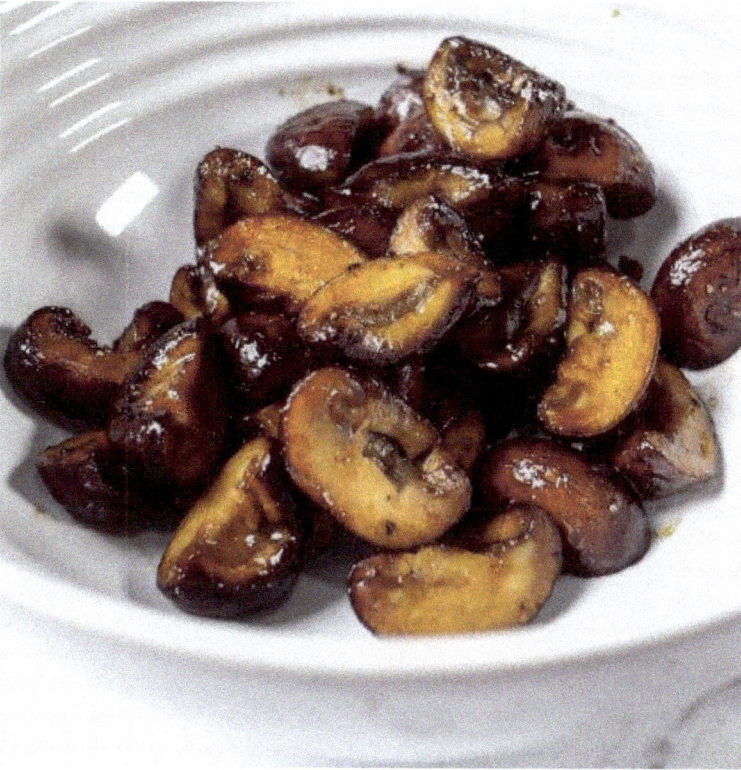

Ingredients

- 2 zucchinis, cut into 1/2-inch slices

- 2 red bell peppers, cut into chunks

- 1/2 pound fresh crimini mushrooms

- 1/2 pound cherry tomatoes

- 1 red onion, cut into 1/2-inch-thick slices

- 1/2 cup olive oil sea salt to taste

- Freshly ground black pepper to taste

Directions:

Preheat your grill for medium-high heat Oil the grate. Mix the zucchinis, green bell peppers, mushrooms, tomatoes, and onion in a bowl. Drizzle some olive oil over vegetables and toss them to coat. Season with sea salt and pepper. Grill the vegetables for 4 minutes per side.

Grilled Asparagus Carrots and Squash Marinade

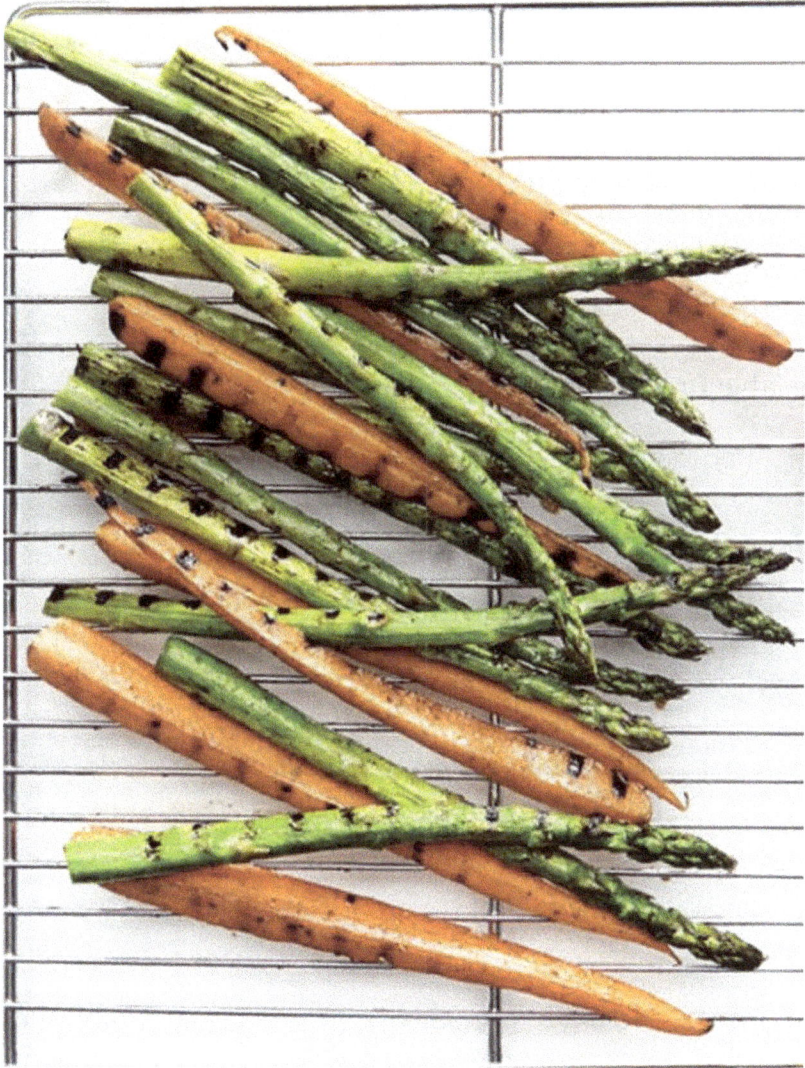

Ingredients

- 1/4 cup extra virgin olive oil

- 2 tablespoons honey

- 4 teaspoons balsamic vinegar

- 1 teaspoon dried oregano

- 1 teaspoon garlic powder

- 1/8 teaspoon rainbow peppercorns

- Sea salt

Vegetable Ingredients

- 1 pound fresh asparagus, trimmed

- 3 small carrots, cut in half lengthwise

- 1 large sweet green pepper, cut into 1-inch strips

- 1 medium yellow summer squash, cut into 1/2-inch slices

- 1 medium yellow onion, cut into wedges

Directions:

Combine the marinade ingredients. Combine the 3 tablespoons marinade and vegetables in a bag.

Marinate 1 1/2 hours at room temperature or overnight in the refrigerator. Grill the vegetables over medium heat for 8-12 minutes or until tender. Sprinkle the remaining marinade.

Grilled Sweet Corns and Portobello

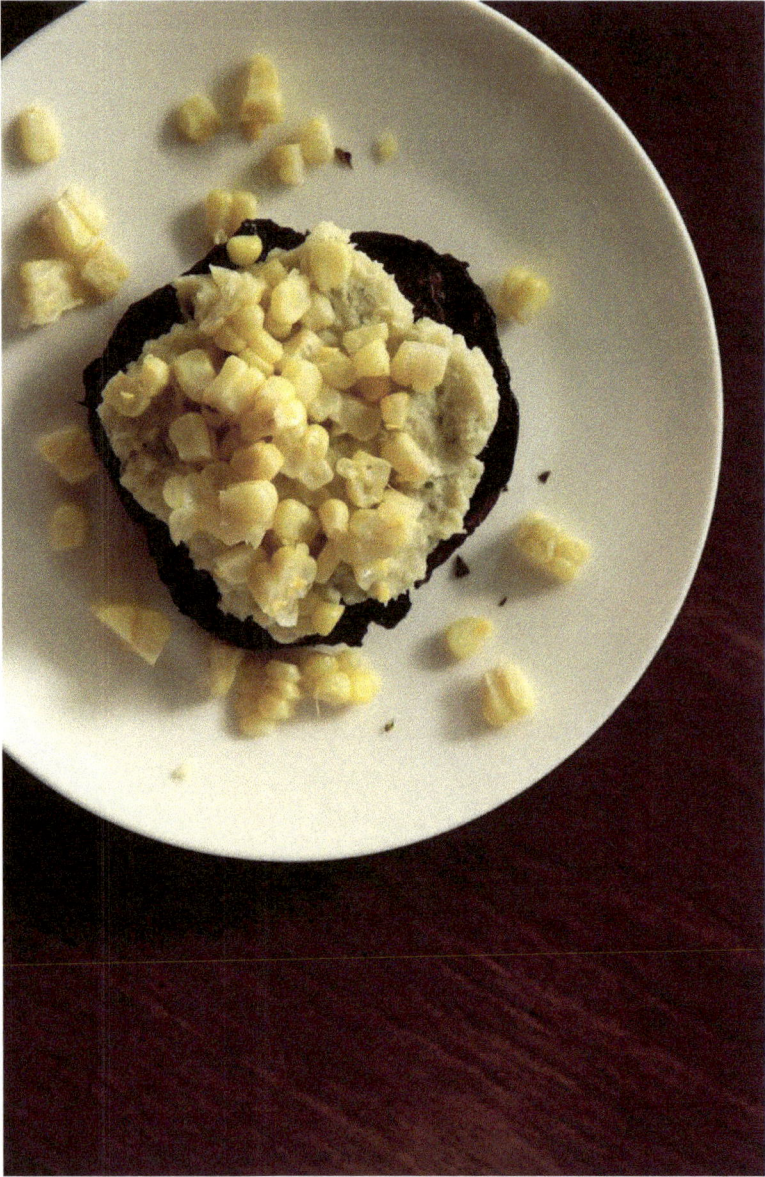

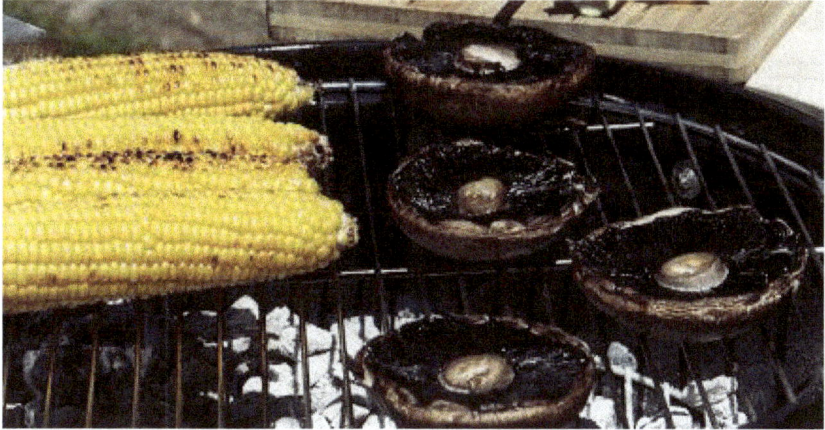

Ingredients

- 2 large Sweet Corns, cut lengthwise

- 5 pcs. Portobello, rinsed and drained

<u>Marinade</u>

- 6 tbsp. extra virgin olive oil

- Sea salt, to taste

- 3 tbsp.distilled white vinegar

- 1 tsp. Dijon mustard

Directions:

Marinate the vegetable with the dressing or marinade ingredients for 15 to 30 min. Grill for 4 minutes over medium heat or until the vegetable becomes tender.

Grilled Bell Pepper and Broccolini

Ingredients

- 2 green Bell Peppers, cut in half

- 10 Broccolini Florets

Marinade Ingredients:

- 6 tbsp. extra virgin olive oil

- Sea salt, to taste

- 3 tbsp. distilled white vinegar

- 1 tsp. sun-dried tomato pesto sauce

Directions:

Marinate the vegctable with the dressing or marinade ingredients for 15 to 30 min. Grill for 4 minutes over medium heat or until the vegetable becomes tender.

Grilled Corn and Crimini Mushrooms

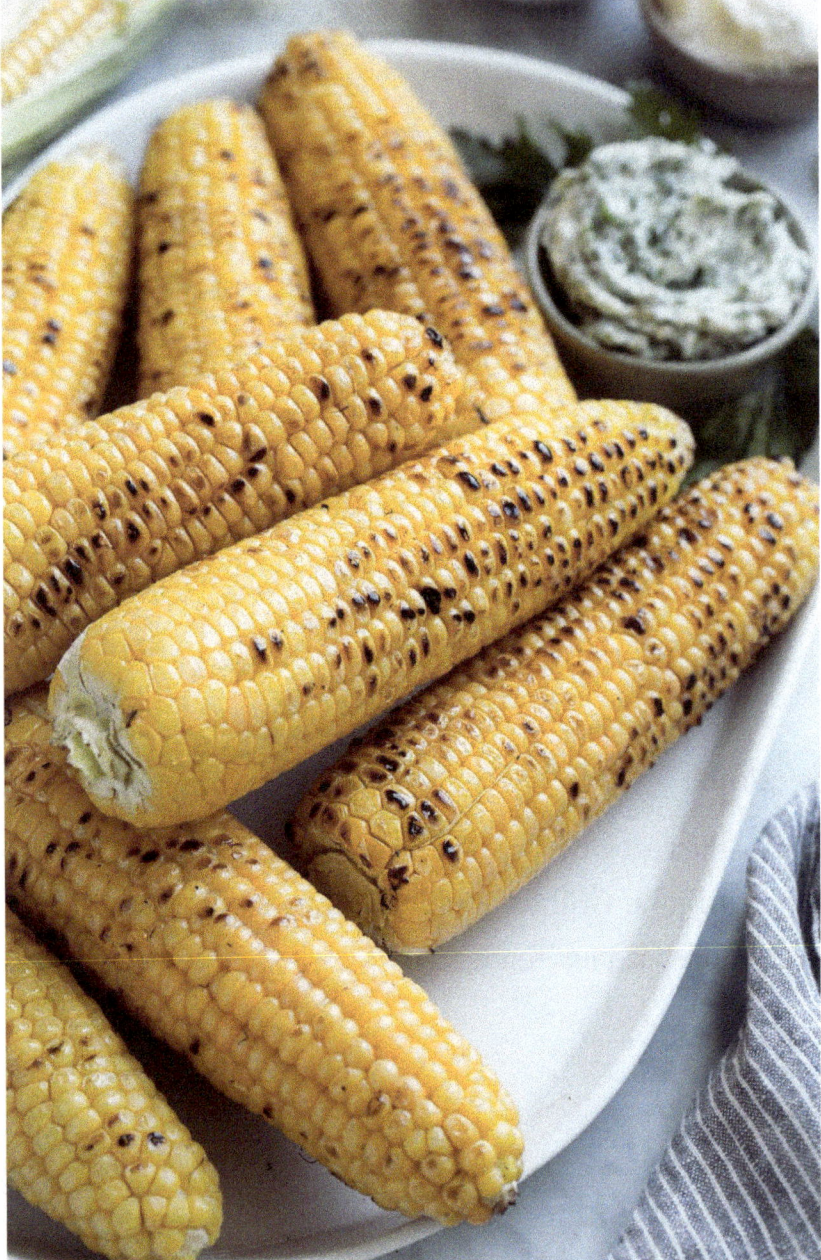

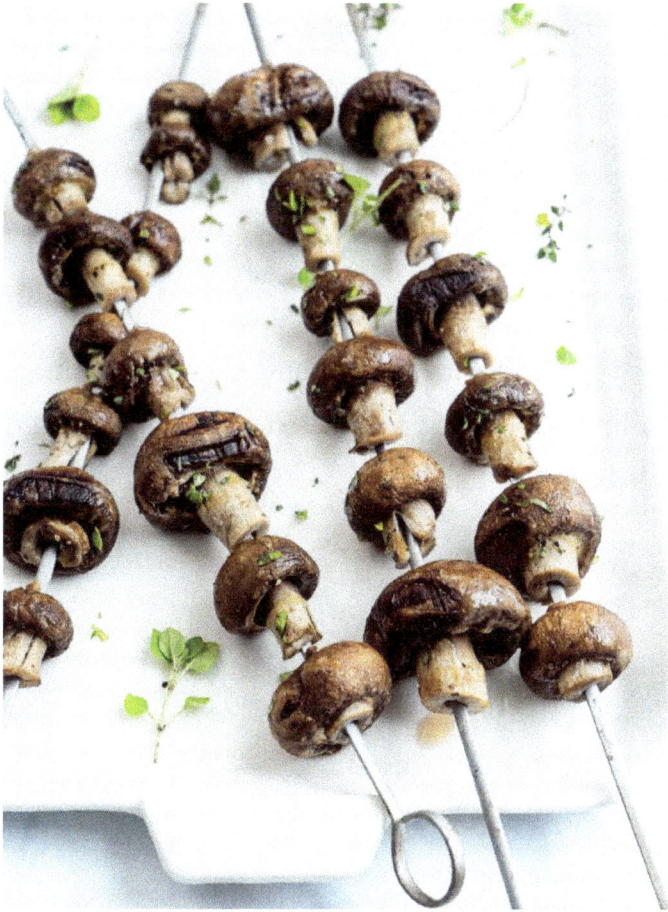

Ingredients

- 2 Corns, cut lengthwise

- 10 Crimini Mushrooms, rinsed and drained

Marinade Ingredients:

- 6 tbsp. extra virgin olive oil

- Sea salt, to taste

- 3 tbsp. distilled white vinegar

- 1 tsp. Dijon mustard

Directions:

Marinate the vegetable with the dressing or marinade ingredients for 15 to 30 min. Grill for 4 minutes over medium heat or until the vegetable becomes tender.

Grilled Zucchini and Pineapple

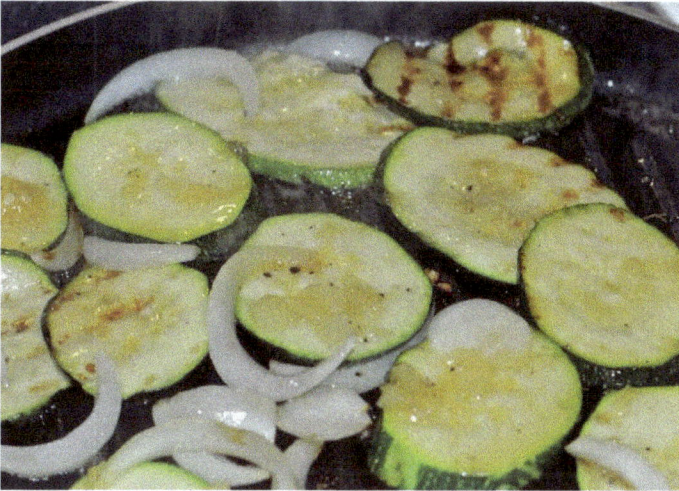

Ingredients

- 2 large zucchini , cut lengthwise into ½ inch slabs

- 2 large red onions, cut into ½ inch rings but don't separate into individual rings

- 1 medium Pineapple, cut into 1/2 inch slices

- 10 Green Beans

Marinade Ingredients:

- 6 tbsp. extra virgin olive oil

- Sea salt, to taste

- 3 tbsp. distilled white vinegar

- 1 tsp. honey

Directions:

Marinate the vegetable with the dressing or marinade ingredients for 15 to 30 min. Grill for 4 minutes over medium heat or until the vegetable becomes tender.

Grilled Asparagus and Mushrooms

Ingredients

- 6 pcs. Crimini mushrooms, rinsed and drained
- 2 pcs. Eggplant, cut lengthwise and cut in half
- 2 pcs. Zucchini, cut lengthwise and cut in half
- 6 pcs. Asparagus

Dressing Ingredients

- 6 tbsp. extra virgin olive oil
- Sea salt, to taste
- 3 tbsp. apple cider vinegar
  1 tbsp. honey
- 1 tsp. Egg-free mayonnaise

Directions:

Marinate the vegetable with the dressing or marinade ingredients for 15 to 30 min. Grill for 4 minutes over medium heat or until the vegetable becomes tender

Grilled Japanese Eggplant Bell Peppers and Broccolini

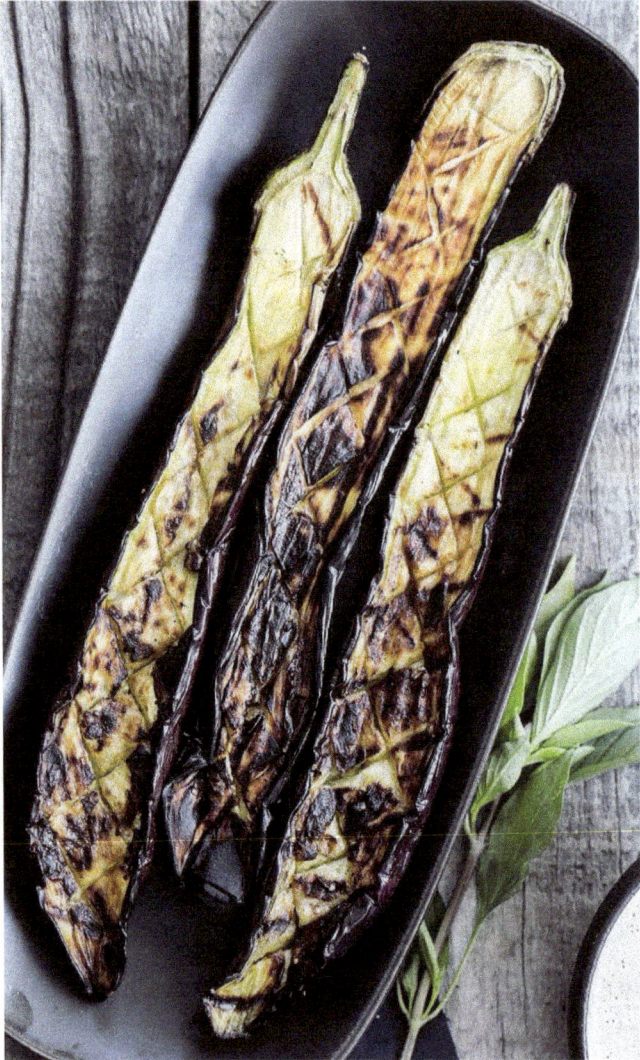

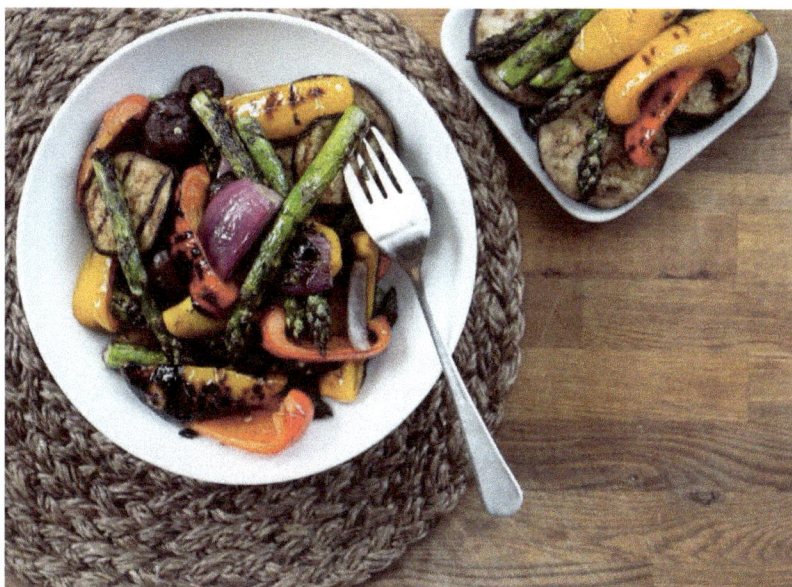

Ingredients

- 2 green Bell Peppers, cut in half

- 10 Broccolini Florets

- 2 pcs. Japanese Eggplant, cut lengthwise and cut in half

Dressing Ingredients

- 6 tbsp. sesame oil

- Sea salt, to taste

- 3 tbsp. distilled white vinegar

- 1 tsp. mayonnaise

Directions:

Marinate the vegetable with the dressing or marinade ingredients for 15 to 30 min. Grill for 4 minutes over medium heat or until the vegetable becomes tender.

Grilled Japanese Bell Pepper and Cauliflower Recipe with Balsamic Glaze

Ingredients

- 2 Yellow Bell Peppers, cut in half lengthwise

- 10 Cauliflower Florets

- 2 pcs. Japanese Eggplant, cut lengthwise and cut in half

<u>Dressing Ingredients</u>

- 6 tbsp. extra virgin olive oil

- Sea salt, to taste

- 3 tbsp. Balsamic vinegar

- 1 tsp. Dijon mustard

Directions:

Marinate the vegetable with the dressing or marinade ingredients for 15 to 30 min. Grill for 4 minutes over medium heat or until the vegetable becomes tender. Grilled Broccoli and Zucchini Recipe Ingredients 2 large Eggplants, cut lengthwise and cut in half 1 large Zucchini, cut lengthwise and cut in half 5

Grilled Eggplant and Yellow Bell Peppers

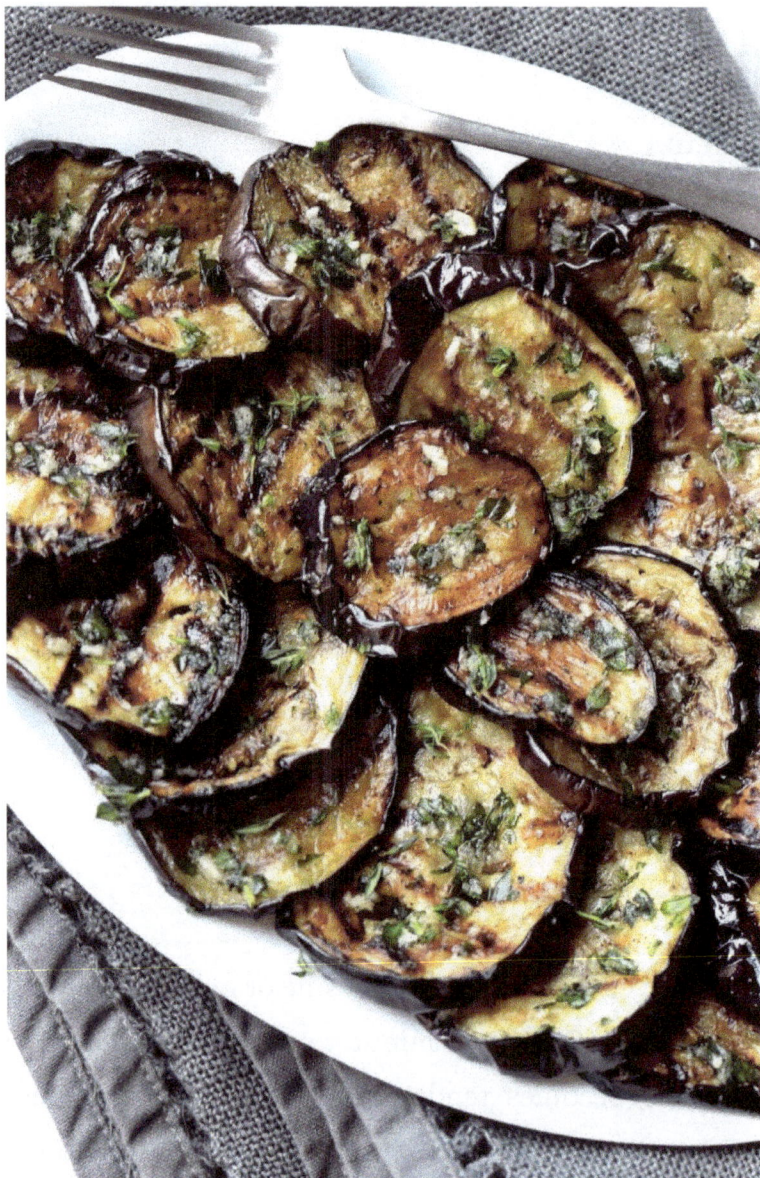

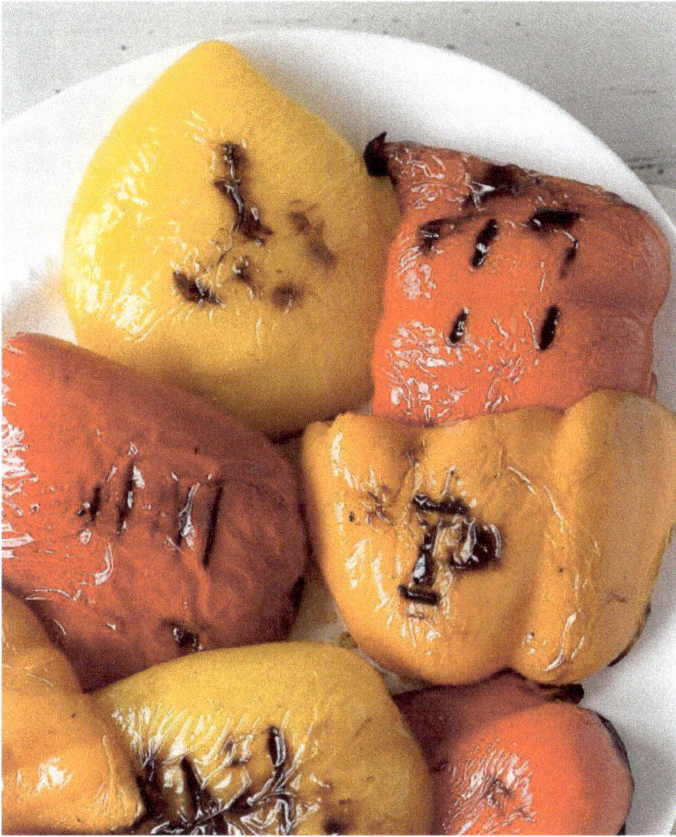

Ingredients

- 2 Yellow Bell Peppers, cut in half

- 10 Broccolini Florets

- 2 pcs. Eggplant, cut lengthwise and cut in half

Dressing Ingredients

- 6 tbsp. olive oil

- Sea salt, to taste

- 3 tbsp. white wine vinegar

- 1 tsp. mustard

Directions:

Marinate the vegetable with the dressing or marinade ingredients for 15 to 30 min. Grill for 4 minutes over medium heat or until the vegetable becomes tender.

Grilled Collard Greens and Portobello Mushrooms

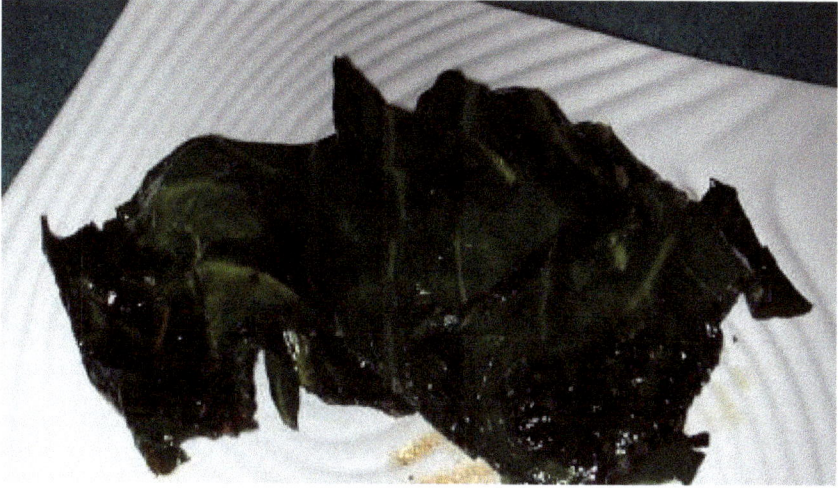

Ingredients

- 1 bunch of collard greens
- 5 pcs. Portobello mushrooms, rinsed and drained
- 10 Asparagus spears

Dressing Ingredients

- 6 tbsp. olive oil
- Sea salt, to taste
- 3 tbsp. white wine vinegar

- 1 tsp. Egg-free mayonnaise

Directions:

Marinate the vegetable with the dressing or marinade ingredients for 15 to 30 min. Grill for 4 minutes over medium heat or until the vegetable becomes tender.

Red Cabbage and Onion in Ranch Dressing

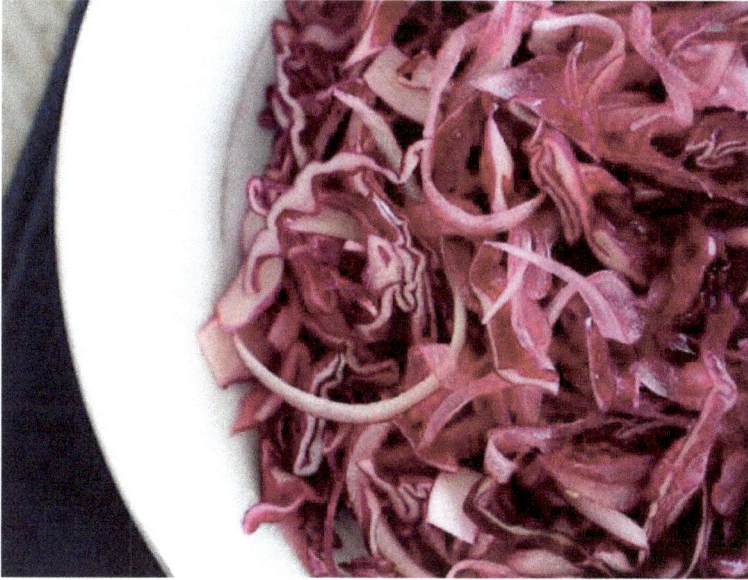

Ingredients

- 1 red cabbage
- 2 large red onions, cut into ½ inch rings but don't separate into individual rings
- 2 tbsp. extra virgin olive oil
- 2 tbsp. ranch dressing mix

Directions:

Marinate the vegetable with the dressing or marinade ingredients for 15 to 30 min. Grill for 4 minutes over medium heat or until the vegetable becomes tender.

Grilled Broccolini Asparagus and Eggplants

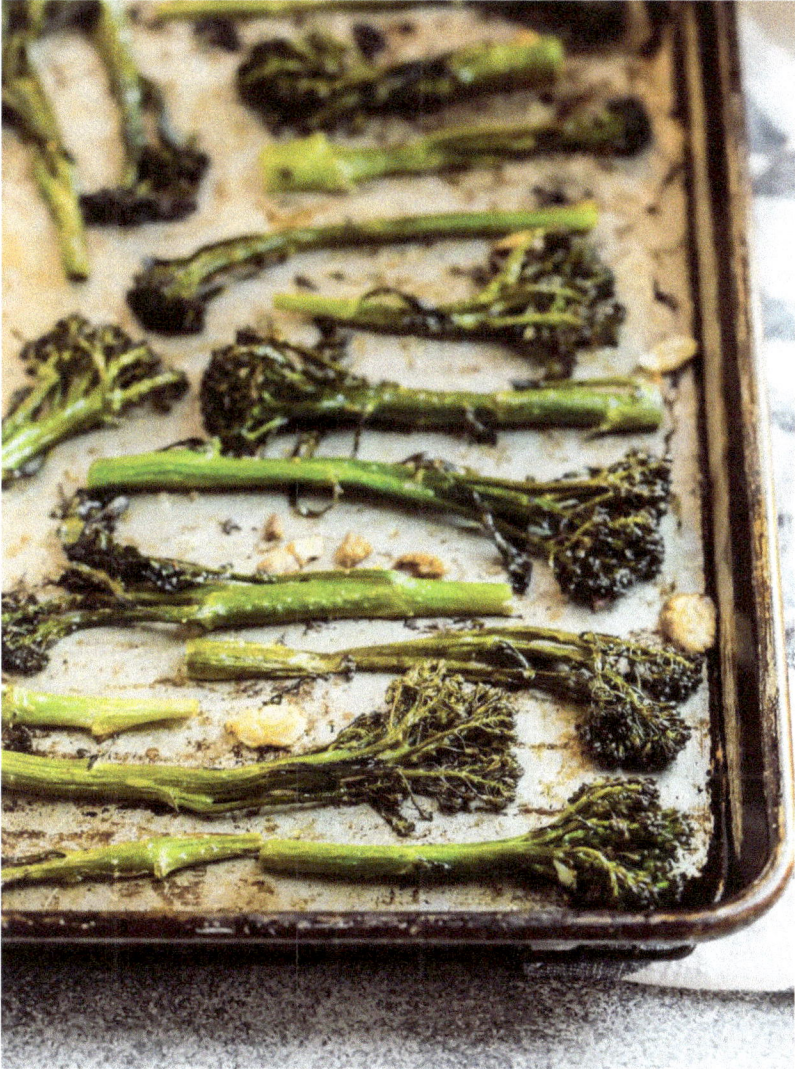

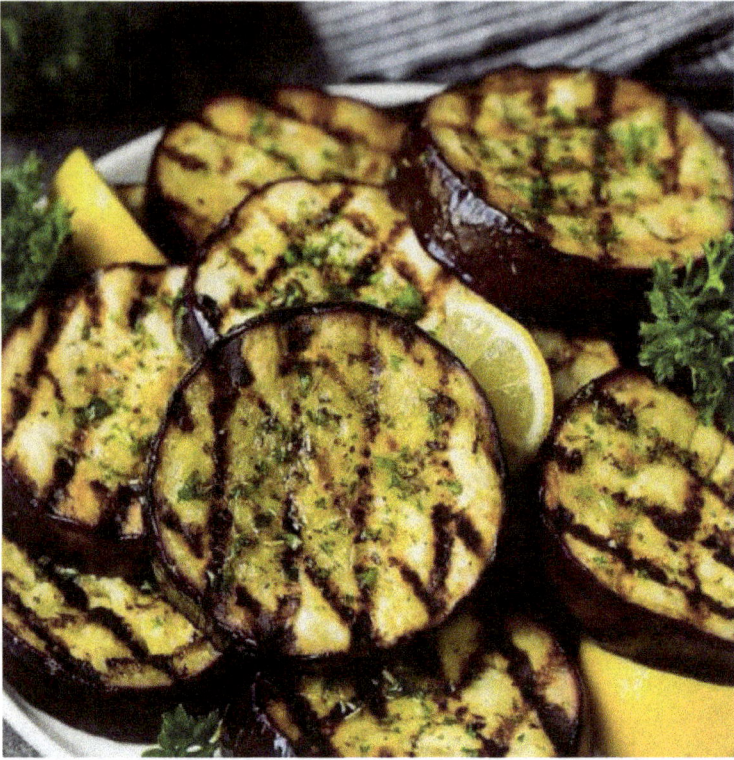

Ingredients

- 1 large Eggplants, cut lengthwise and cut in half

- 1 bunch of turnip greens

- 10 Asparagus spears

- 10 Broccolini Florets

Marinade Ingredients:

- 6 tbsp. extra virgin olive oil

- Sea salt, to taste 3 tbsp.

- distilled white vinegar

- 1 tsp. Dijon mustard

Directions:

Marinate the vegetable with the dressing or marinade ingredients for 15 to 30 min. Grill for 4 minutes over medium heat or until the vegetable becomes tender.

Grilled Rutabaga and Mustard Greens

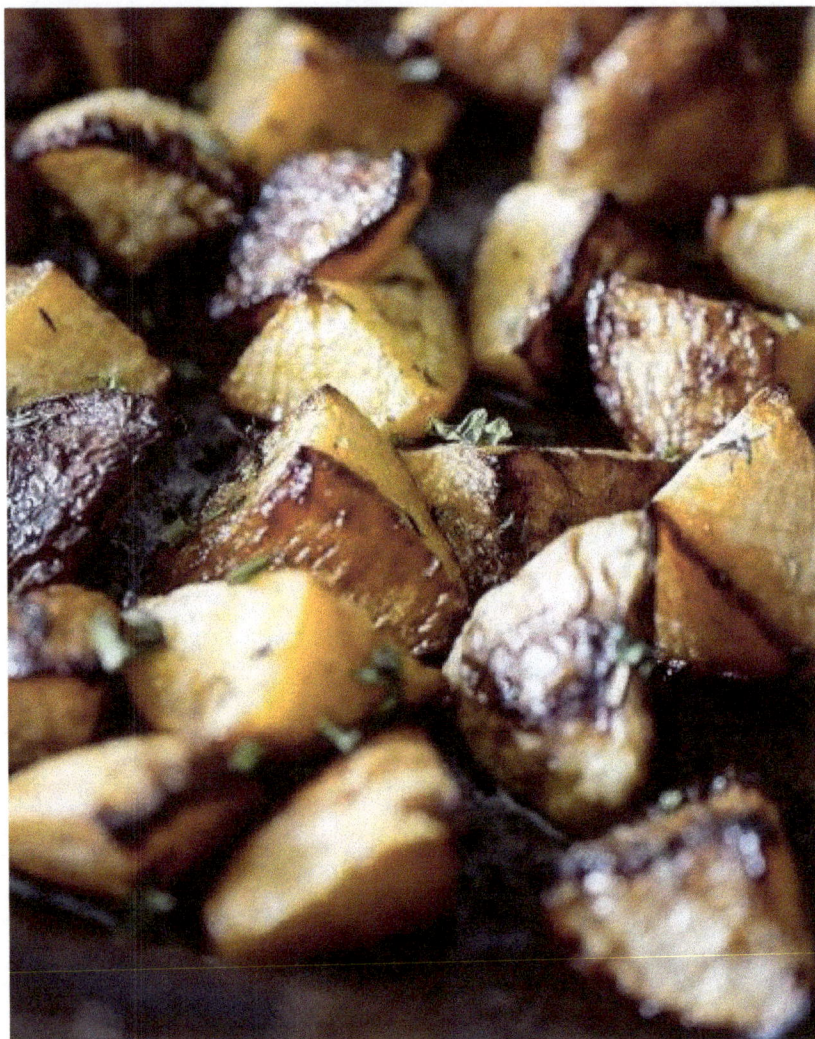

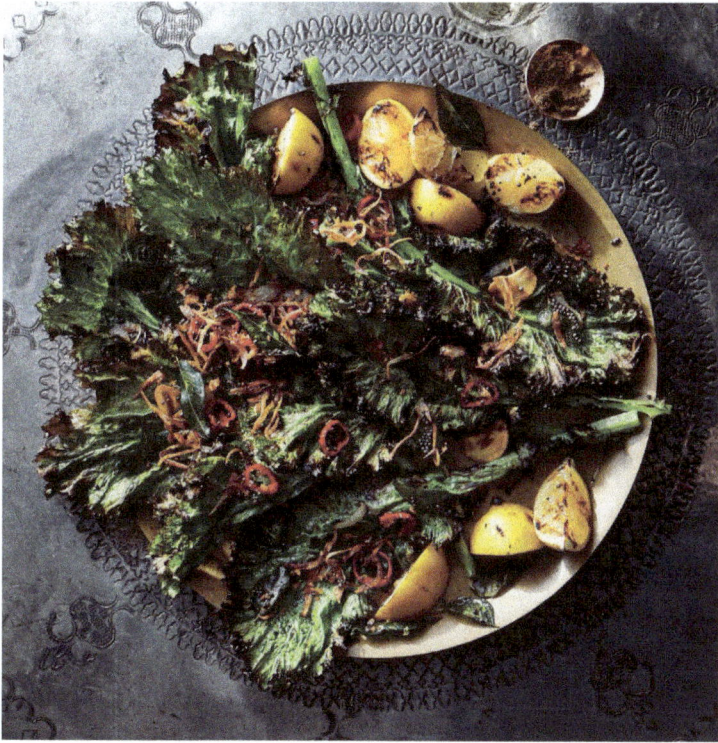

Ingredients

- 1 medium Rutabaga, peeled and cut in half lengthwise

- 1 large red onion, cut into ½ inch rings but don't separate into individual rings

- 1 bunch of mustard greens

Dressing Ingredients

- 6 tbsp. olive oil

- Sea salt, to taste

- 3 tbsp. white wine vinegar

- 1 tsp. English mustard

Directions:

Marinate the vegetable with the dressing or marinade ingredients for 15 to 30 min. Grill for 4 minutes over medium heat or until the vegetable becomes tender.

Grilled Turnips with Broccoli

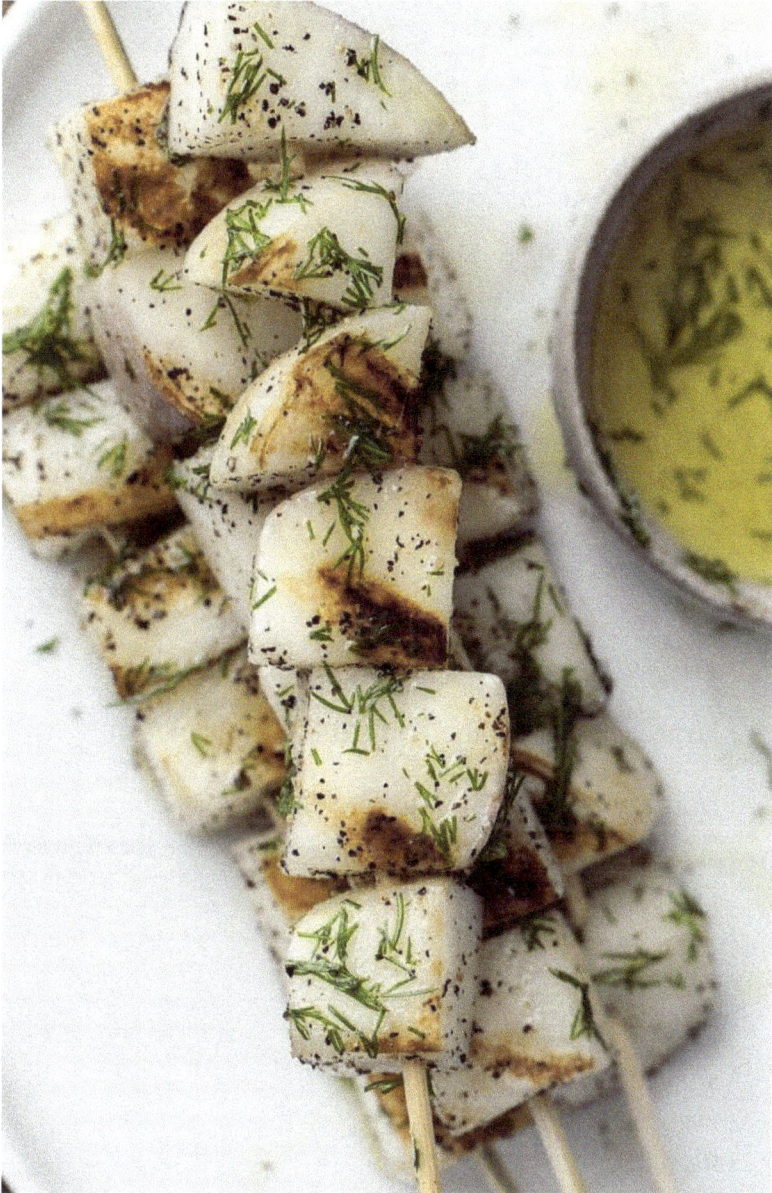

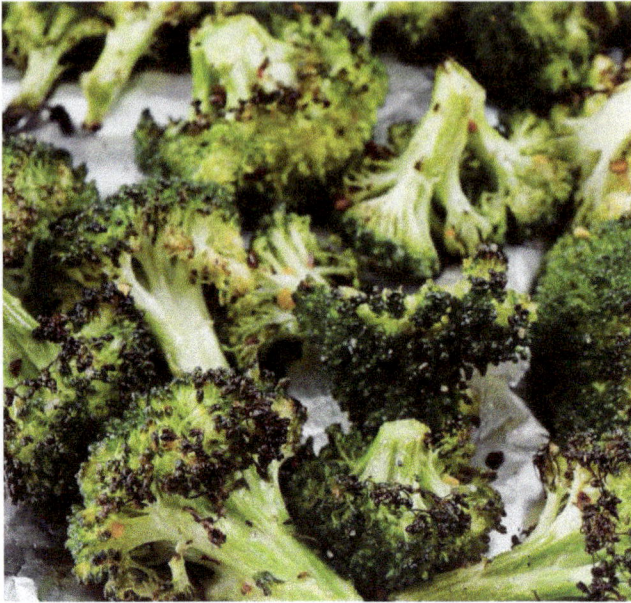

Ingredients

- 10 Broccoli florets

- 1 large turnips, peeled and cut lengthwise

- 1 red cabbage, cut in half

Dressing Ingredients

- 6 tbsp. olive oil

- Sea salt, to taste

- 3 tbsp. white wine vinegar

- 1 tsp. Egg-free mayonnaise

Directions:

Marinate the vegetable with the dressing or marinade ingredients for 15 to 30 min. Grill for 4 minutes over medium heat or until the vegetable becomes tender.

Lightning Source UK Ltd.
Milton Keynes UK
UKHW020718270521
384465UK00005B/213

9 781802 695717